Relationship Therapy

Relationship Therapy

A therapist's tale

Rosie March-Smith

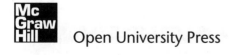

Open University Press

Open University Press
McGraw-Hill Education
McGraw-Hill House
Shoppenhangers Road
Maidenhead
Berkshire
England
SL6 2QL

email: enquiries@openup.co.uk
world wide web: www.openup.co.uk

and Two Penn Plaza, New York, NY 10121–2289, USA

First published 2011

A catalogue record of this book is available from the British Library

ISBN: 978-0-33-523892-7 (pb) 978-0-33-523893-4 (hb)
eISBN: 978-0-33-523894-1

Library of Congress Cataloging-in-Publication Data
CIP data applied for

Typeset by RefineCatch Limited, Bungay, Suffolk
Printed in the UK by Bell and Bain Ltd, Glasgow

Fictitious names of companies, products, people, characters and/or data that may be used herein (in case studies or in examples) are not intended to represent any real individual, company, product or event.

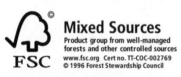

Mixed Sources
Product group from well-managed
forests and other controlled sources
www.fsc.org   Cert no. TT-COC-002769
© 1996 Forest Stewardship Council

The McGraw·Hill Companies

For D.R.S.

This beautifully written and accessible book will be of considerable value to many. Therapists, trainees and those who are simply interested in how and why we relate the way we do, will find gems in this book. Its richness lies in the weaving of theory and personal testimony in a truly integrative and fascinating way.

Dr Moira Walker

Contents

Acknowledgements

When I was researching this book, that old instinct for a story once so useful as a journalist, luckily came back to serve me again. Men and women appeared from their world, often thousands of miles apart, carrying rich seams of material for the mining. For instance, 'Lara' I met in a mountain village in Majorca, whence she had fled to recover from a long relationship breakdown back home in Seattle. In a series of emails later, she provided me with valuable insight into the insidious impact of living with a sociopath.

Then there was a chance meeting with Darla Franey in a busy French hotel foyer, and within minutes we had discovered a common interest in counselling and psychotherapy. This resulted in her sending later a moving account of her work with traumatized Afro-American youngsters in California. Helen Derek, an old colleague from newspaper days, flew in from Japan after many years' absence, got back in touch just when I was writing about the power of the mind – and produced her extraordinary tale.

My thanks to them, and to the many other new and old friends who were also happy to be interviewed, telling their stories so openly, willing to share their experiences. For obvious reasons of confidentiality they cannot be named, although I should have dearly liked to acknowledge them publicly for their gift to us all. But they know who they are. I am indebted to them for their true generosity of spirit.

In Relate's Barbara Bloomfield I found a warm and ready spokesperson to provide professional gravitas to the concluding chapters, as also happened with Dr Rich Hycner, a Gestalt psychotherapist from the United States who permitted me to quote him at length during his visit to a West Country seminar. To Dr Moira Walker and Professor Michael Jacobs I owe a profound debt of gratitude for their encouragement and support. My thanks also to Open University Press editor Dr Monika Lee, and to her unfailingly helpful team.

This book would literally not have been written without the patient technical instruction given by my son, James, who – with his brother, Matt, providing invaluable back-up at other times – managed to keep me (much more used to typewriters than information technology) this side of sanity when the computer gave trouble. Heartfelt thanks to them both.

Foreword

We have long expanded Descartes' definition of personal existence – 'I think therefore I am' – but I could not help thinking of it as I started to read Rosie March-Smith's book. I knew that I wanted to replace 'think' with 'relate' to describe her theme as I understood it, although I did not like the phrase that resulted: 'I relate, therefore I am'. For a start it sounds ugly when spoken, but my reservation was more than that. How could I account for the solitary, schizoid person who appears unable to relate to other people, but clearly has a self, and a personal existence? He or she surely 'is'? But of course that is the case. Such a person relates still, even if narrowly, to himself or herself, or to non-human objects. Relates he or she still does, and so any relationship is essential for survival.

Relatedness, that is the key. I, and you the reader, need relatedness – so much broader a term than 'relationship', although relationship therapy is obviously the aim of this book. Relatedness, as well as relationship, is what Rosie demonstrates so clearly throughout this book. She begins by demonstrating just how much our present attitudes, wishes, fears and behaviours can be dictated by unrecognized forces within us – the force of past experience, the compulsion of unconscious material to respond to situations that are in fact not new, but repetitions of what we have already been through. This is Freud's 'return of the repressed', or Winnicott's accurate observation that fear of a breakdown now is not of a new experience, but of one that has already happened, often long ago. 'There are moments, according to my experience, when a patient needs to be told that the breakdown, a fear of which destroys his or her life, has already been. It is a fact that is carried round hidden away in the unconscious' (1974: 104).

Let me continue my term 'relatedness'. What is particularly impressive is the way that Rosie relates (both in the sense of 'tells' and of 'joins up') different therapeutic theories and practices to each other – she can draw upon a variety of ways of understanding or reaching or working with buried material. Hers is a superb example of how an integrative practitioner is able to relate one approach to another with ease. It is rare to find citations from so many different perspectives, yet this is no eclectic mish-mash, but a careful relating of ideas, a subtle weaving of the insights of practitioner authors into her text, showing the relevance of their work and the relatedness of their words to her themes. But what makes Rosie's writing special is that she is just as ready to interview those whose stories and experiences have not been published, and that she reports their original words as much as she quotes from established sources.

Relating the ordinary person and the professional communicator makes for a blend that is particularly refreshing and is so clearly relevant to her themes.

One aspect of this is the way Rosie highlights the relatedness of the different parts of ourselves. Of course it is important to pay full attention to relatedness to other people, but it is equally true that we need to relate as fully as we can to the different aspects of ourselves – call them subpersonalities, or internal objects, or what you will, this necessity for the parts of our inner world to interrelate is highlighted in what she writes. At the same time she shows the relevance of the internal for outward relationships, as the chapter on couples work illustrates. She goes on to make particular reference to Asperger's Syndrome and how this can affect a couple – a unique feature in a book of this nature. She also adds, in the chapter after that, an extremely important theme, that is the way one generation is related in more than the obvious sense to the generation(s) above and the generation(s) that will follow. Relatedness is everywhere of course, and this is what the therapist needs to recognize in its many and varied dimensions.

It goes without saying that the way therapist and client relate to each other lies at the heart of the therapeutic enterprise. The years of experience that Rosie has as a therapist are clear from her range of examples, but more than that there is an obvious care in her interventions which illustrates her capacity for relatedness to her clients. Connections abound, and relatedness needs thinking about. Descartes may not have got the whole picture when thinking about personal identity, but thinking certainly is part of relating. Chapter 7 shows how important it is to think about and then challenge assumptions. And this is a thoughtful book.

Nor do I forget that the verb 'relate' can also mean telling a story. Rosie's talent as a writer shines through in the ease with which the reader will turn the pages, because she relates her stories well. This is a book that, as I read, not only reminds me of much that I have known but perhaps given less emphasis to than it deserved; but which prompted me to reflect that this is not just a book for student therapists and for seasoned practitioners, but one which will be readily accessible to many clients and to the interested wider public.

These distinct features about this book require one further relatedness, since there is never just one strand which needs to be followed in order to see how relationships function. The facets of relationships that are discussed in each of the eight chapters are also related to each other, in a complex web of relatedness. I have in the past described this as a type of cat's cradle – that weaving of string patterns that we once learned in childhood. The cat's cradle, where it functions well, holds these different facets in a creative tension. But let one part of the cradle slip and the cradle will fall. Unconscious influences, subpersonalities, the legacy of parent–child relationships, thought patterns, emotional responsiveness, histories and family myths, all these and more go to make up the way we relate to each other; and, indeed, are influenced by each string of the web.

Michael Jacobs

Preface

Relationship difficulties are talked about every day: in the workplace, college, pubs, locker rooms, on holiday, and in the bedroom. Nobody would deny that this is a sad reflection of our times. If current trends persist, nearly half of the marriages in Britain will end in divorce, representing the highest rate of marital breakdown in Europe; the figure is even higher in the United States. We can only guess at the comparable numbers of unmarried couples who split up, the breakdown casualties including gay, lesbian and bisexual pairs. So why do so many relationships fail? What is really going on when love turns to despair?

Men and women believe they fell in love with the right partner, chosen with varying degrees of care for a long-term significant time together. Yet, clearly, for many it all goes disastrously wrong, with the underlying cause unrecognized and usually unexplored. Relationships mostly fail because either or both partners are living in a continuum of unresolved childhood issues. It is these issues which cloud choice, which drive couples to find themselves in multiple crises, baffled and hurt by the behaviour of their mate and seemingly unable to make sense of any part of it. It is also these unresolved issues which influence much of their interaction with everyone else.

This book is concerned not only with couples: relationship difficulties occur across the human spectrum – siblings, children, parents, colleagues, and so on – and will continue to manifest through those unresolved childhood issues if left unchecked. The degree of upset they cause usually determines why people seek professional help; and it is often a crisis which nudges that process to start.

As an integrative psychotherapist I have worked for 20 years with clients individually (usually in relationships) and also with couples presenting relationship problems. Most, however, struggle unaware with the impact of long-forgotten childhood lacks. This struggle is evident in their outward confusion and despair. Yet the driving force behind this state of affairs lies with their unconscious 'controllers', those split-off aspects of themselves, out of touch with the adult self and protected from further hurt by functioning from their 'frozen in time' child viewpoint. They make up secret dramatis personae who wield such enormous power from the inner world that they can ruin a partnership, sabotage closeness with offspring or siblings, push away love and friendship, and most importantly affect the relationship with self.

These hidden controllers have the ultimate hold on the fabric or quality of all our relationships if they are left undiscovered and not reintegrated into the psyche. They operate throughout the day and night, reacting to triggers unwittingly pulled by others, or by their own thought processes. Only when the extent of this hold is realized can a glimmer of understanding open the way: here lies the key task for counsellors and psychotherapists.

Their clients will need commitment to be prepared to tread unknown territory, with no certain way out. They may also have to contend with the cynicism of a partner. They must summon up a certain amount of courage too, because accepting that they have hidden parts of themselves functioning unrecognized through everyday behaviour is an alarming nettle to grasp. They will also need an ability to reflect upon what they learn, to make connections and consciously start to identify how and when the dramatis personae make their appearance. This, then, might be the time when a new emotional frame begins for them.

Unpacking the layers

Numerous research studies have shown that nearly three-quarters of the mind remains hidden – leaving about a quarter to run our daily lives. In times of psychological crisis that segment is usually inadequate on its own to go down to the remaining areas for answers, classically achieved through analysis. Slowly unpacking the layers buried in the unconscious realms has been the traditional clinical route taken for well over a century. However, classical analysis valuable though it unquestionably is, can be lengthy and expensive.

There are other methods (largely based on the tenets of the analytical approach) which integrative colleagues and I have found to be effective in our overstretched society. These more eclectic approaches support the theme of this book: that of discovering the core issues within a relatively brief time, and the absolute necessity for looking backwards. One could say it is less the fruit, more the root which should concern us. This contention will perhaps seem outdated by some of the newer disciplines in the therapeutic arena: cognitive behaviour therapy (CBT) being one example, whose tenets focus more on problem solving in the present.

Although praised as a tool and one favoured by the National Health Service for its clear-cut working model requiring patients to make lists and do homework, CBT is not the panacea that was anticipated. As David Edwards and Michael Jacobs point out in their book *Conscious and Unconscious* (2003: 90): 'A. Hackmann remarks that "focusing on the first thoughts that come up may miss much of the meaning of an upsetting event . . . we need to tackle both the surface weeds (negative automatic thoughts, images etc.) and the deeper 'roots' (underlying beliefs and assumptions) of the meanings we give to events" (1997: 125–6).'

When I began in practice it was quite usual to see clients for several years at a stretch. Now, a seamless shift has occurred in that the demand for brief therapy, particularly in emergency casework, has thrown into sharp perspective the fact that core issues do appear soon, often within the first few hours, and should no longer be left on the back burner for deeper exploration months down the line. This is not to suggest the latter approach is wrong, far from it; analysis is both elegant and fascinating and deservedly continues in eminence. Yet useful work can be achieved within a remarkably short time frame. If the root cause becomes obvious soon it is certainly possible, even within a limited period only, to achieve satisfactory insight on both sides. Has some psychological osmosis come about in the twenty-first century which accelerates – even invites – swifter interventions these days? Case studies introduced later may better illustrate the point.

Down the generations

Our first relationship is with our parents, or carers, and if they experienced lacks in their childhood, their own parenting having been given mixed or painful messages, then it is likely we suffered lacks too. Never being able, for example, to predict mother's or father's mood, striving to keep the peace at home no matter what it took (usually compliance or, for some personality types, emotional freezing) will have inexorably laid down the markers for degrees of dysfunctional behaviour in the future. Generation after generation inherit the pattern, as Richard Madeley describes in his biography *Fathers & Sons* (2009), discussed in Chapter 6.

If we were fortunate instead to inherit more aware parenting, then we might have been gently steered away from our over-willingness to please; encouraged to voice our negative feelings without dread of punishment, and carefully protected from humiliation. Should we have been among the lucky few, basking in 'good enough mothering', as defined by psychoanalyst Donald Winnicott in his *Home Is Where We Start From* (1986: 144), we might even have been supported to express the whole range of feelings where appropriate, to learn when to control the more tempestuous kind, and taught how to move confidently into the outside world without fear; where consideration for others prevents us from causing harm and our willingness to please comes not from dread but from love.

Most of us dread exclusion: we need to be included in the pack. In primitive societies our survival literally depended upon this. Alone, we would perish. As Will Schutz says in his book *Joy*: 'It is likely that this basic fear of abandonment or isolation is the most potent of all interpersonal fears' (1967: 136). This basic fear of rejection drives us to forge acceptable false selves to present to the outer world, confining our unacceptable selves to the darker corners of our inner world. These split-off parts have a tendency to reappear at some point in our lives, either insidiously or in volcanic-like eruptions. Healing lies in understanding why unconsciously we needed once to split off those parts, so often concerning faulty relationships, directly or indirectly.

When new clients exclaim: 'This is a light bulb moment! Now I begin to see what all this is about' then there is real possibility that their distress or confusion will clear; perhaps for the benefit too of future generations. With earlier clients' generous cooperation in sharing here (years later) some of the details of their own 'light bulb' moments, I offer the following chapters, with their anonymized case studies and follow-up interviews, hopefully to show how excavation work in psychological therapies can and does flick the switch to illuminate relationship breakdown.

1 Powerful hidden controllers

It is a widely held view nowadays that a huge proportion of our mind lies hidden. Like the iceberg that shows only its tip, the unconscious takes up two-thirds of the total – and sometimes appears as treacherous as an iceberg. It can also be a beautiful ally, a bewitching friend who seems to know all the answers once we have learned how to ask the questions, sometimes when we cannot. It delivers through dreams, images, hunches, feelings, memories, a vast store of material comparable in its ability to a highly sophisticated computer. It tells our body how to work, it reminds us of urgent tasks we had forgotten, it files away a record of everything we have ever done, or felt.

As if this were not impressive enough, despite the randomness with which our mysterious realms seem to operate, quantum physicist John Hagelin tells us (2006): 'We are using at most five per cent of the *potential* of the human mind' (my italics). And yet, like the treacherous iceberg, this powerful, creative mind can sink our hopes of happiness with bewildering force. How can this conflicting state of affairs be explained? Why does one person access the depths of his psyche, yet another flounder? For the present, and until the scope of our human potential is somehow revealed, we are in a state of unknowing.

However, we do know that fear and insecurity are two primary factors that will usually account for unpleasant, negative control from the unconscious. It is this understanding which can take today's practitioner into comparatively familiar waters to work productively with clients, aiming (just as the early pioneers did) to grasp the meaning of the hidden controllers when they assert their influence. But beyond interesting glimpses of the much more benign control from hidden realms, we are still powerless to tap or discover more of the mysteries of the human mind. Given that psychotherapy began a century ago, we may have to wait another hundred years to discover what riches lie below the surface of our minds, and how we might contact them at will.

In the meantime, using what information we do have, we might start by outlining some unusual case studies and take a brief glance at the extraordinary diversity of phenomena which the unconscious mind has already demonstrated to some clients in my consulting room. Some of the material is immediately relevant to counselling or psychotherapy; some is not, certainly not at first sight. However, we should at least concede the sheer complexity which lies beneath the surface of our minds, whether we liken their domain to icebergs, seabeds, islands, or roots in the earth – and acknowledge the weight of importance such clues imply.

CASE STUDY
A problem at the office

Leo, a business consultant, began to realize he was needing to rush to the lavatory too many times during meetings, their varying levels of importance strangely linked with his bladder needs. The problem got so bad that Leo sought therapeutic help. 'I'm getting panic attacks too,' he said ruefully, 'and these are even worse to deal with because they happen when I'm driving to work as well as in the office. I realize these attacks and the weak bladder control are all about stress, but they are ruining my chances of promotion. I worry that colleagues might begin to doubt my stability. And all this is seriously affecting my marriage – my wife cannot understand what has got into me, and why I'm not man enough to conquer my fears.'

As we explored his current and earlier life experiences, a picture emerged of his never having had much confidence; a high achiever academically, but anxious and shy in social settings. Bullying at school had been unpleasant and frightening, but he stoically got through his education and went on to university to earn a good degree. A few years later he married, and Leo seemed content enough with his new life, if a little worried he could afford to keep up the large payments on his first ever mortgage.

When pressure in the office intensified demands Leo began to dread demotion, or worse, because of poor performance. The prospect of public humiliation (job loss or peer jokes) was an additional burden he struggled with constantly, although so far no one at work had made any comment. His panic attacks were growing in ferocity. He even began taking incontinence pads to wear in the office. Agoraphobia became another problem: he was afraid to go to the supermarket for fear of being in big open spaces. He was also afraid of being caught out at the checkout, in front of a long line of customers, and needing to abandon his trolley to run for the toilets. His wife despaired of him ever becoming a reliable companion and mate. At this point, Leo was ready to try psychotherapy.

By the second session, we talked about his childhood. Yes, there had been a bit of bed-wetting (his parents were quite strict and he was a sensitive little boy), but this area felt unproductive in our work because wetting had been overcome within a normal time. It seemed more likely that the trauma was connected with the unexpected in Leo's young life, perhaps where an emergency call of nature embarrassed him greatly.

'Think of outside activities, play or sport, perhaps: does any memory come up that involved you needing to pee when it wasn't a good idea? Wetting your pants when you were out with Mum and Dad – maybe they were cross with you? Imagine the fear, if you badly wanted to go and couldn't because there was no loo nearby.' Leo suddenly had the answer. He looked astounded, as the long-forgotten episode suddenly popped into his head, 30 years later and hidden away until acute stress steered him to therapy and released the lock.

> **66** It was the school pantomime! I was five, and playing the part of Peter Pan, in those leggings and tunic. I must have been so nervous being on stage, I wet myself big time: apparently I dripped on to the stage and there was a big damp stain down my leggings. The audience roared with laughter, though I was too humiliated and upset to register they were probably sympathetic. What really hurt was my parents later telling the rest of the family how funny it had been. And that wasn't the end of it, either. They'd tell other people in my hearing, and they always laughed, I suppose because it was presented to them as hilarious. My experience was quite the opposite, so I was very confused.
>
> (personal communication) **99**

This proved the core to the present trouble, one which was reached in a few hours' therapy sessions. Leo reported (in the remaining weeks we both felt he needed in order to consolidate his new-found self-confidence) that his panic attacks had melted away, that his need to take comfort breaks had reduced to a normal level, and that agoraphobia no longer troubled him. He called me a year later, still reporting the same good news. Most importantly, his self-esteem and obvious work confidence had earned him promotion, not the sack.

His marriage had taken on new dimensions, for not only was Leo 'more of a man, a bigger man' as he proudly recalled his wife commenting, but he was finding his relationship with her had somehow benefited from his new insights. She was readier than ever before to talk and own her feelings of occasional inadequacy and under-confidence. His therapy sessions had spilled over into the partnership in a way neither of us had anticipated.

Here we have an illustration of the hidden controller sending up distress signals because the pressure in his external world had powerful 'on stage' resonance: that of the threat, the dread of humiliation. Those dormant painful memories needed to appear because they had begun seriously to affect his life.

At first it seemed to Leo that a demonic presence was taking him over. Sigmund Freud knew about this. He had this to say in the 1920s: 'Cases of demoniacal possession correspond to the neuroses of the present day. What in those days were thought to be evil spirits to us are base and evil wishes, the derivatives of impulses which have been rejected and repressed' (1923b: 436–72).

Accompanying guide

We have a more recent – and compelling – view from post-Jungian analyst James Hillman, who describes our demons as daimons, as did Plato and the Greeks, when they were referring to heart, spirit, or the soul. Hillman, author of *The Soul's Code*, tells us that Plato believed the soul chooses its particular destiny, guarded by a daimon ever since birth, 'venerable, articulate, complete', and that it acts as an accompanying guide who remembers its calling. Hillman goes on to say:

> 66 The daimon's 'reminders' work in many ways. The daimon motivates. It protects. It invents and persists with stubborn fidelity. It resists compromising reasonableness and often forces deviance and oddity upon its keeper, especially when it is neglected or opposed. It offers comfort and can pull you into its shell, but cannot abide innocence. It can make the body ill. It is out of step with time, finding all sorts of faults, gaps and knots in the flow of life – and it prefers them. It has affinities with myth, since it is itself a mythical being and thinks in mythical patterns. The daimon has prescience . . . not perfect, but limited to the significance of the life in which it has embodiment.
>
> (1996: 39–40) 99

And so it could be said that Leo's daimon or demon was appropriately using the work pressures to force him to address his repressed underlying problem. Never before in his adult life had those pressures been urgent enough to release the dread into consciousness. Leo's existence until then was exactly that: merely existing. He got by without much joy or satisfaction, yet acceptable enough to convince himself he was reasonably happy. Today, however, he is a contented, truly fulfilled man and his real happiness is obvious.

Because we do not ourselves yet know how to command the human mind to create these necessary healing changes (reintegrating the split-off parts) at home, or spontaneously present essential memories to provide the answers, therapists and counsellors are more than ever urgently needed to help the increasing numbers of breakdown and stress-related mental illnesses presented in GP surgeries and in private consulting rooms. Their job is to work in cooperation with the psyche, as if in joint effort to free the controllers from their self-imposed prison, opening the way to a more balanced, whole emotional life.

But sometimes our social conditioning convinces us that little problems in the past are insignificant; we are, after all, adult now, men and women who pass examinations and secure mortgages. 'How can decades ago when we were little have any bearing on the present day?' people ask. I never fail to wonder at this attitude: exemplified, interestingly, particularly by worldly professionals like bank managers, engineers, scientists or lawyers, accustomed to working with the left hemisphere of their brain (the right side concerned with non-linear thinking), and who seem tenaciously to hold this dismissive view.

Pride and fear of humiliation can lie behind resistance in many would-be clients. Only when a major jolt, such as redundancy from their high-powered job, brings them into the therapy room, sometimes under guise of post traumatic stress disorder (a socially acceptable, modern condition often mentioned in connection with raids, terrorist attacks, war-shocked soldiers) do they feel they can justify their reluctant stance. Then they become so fascinated by the unfolding story from their inner world, and the feeling of well-being their insight gives, that they often change their opinion about the value of looking back.

CASE STUDY

Trapped in the dark

This was the case with Sarah, a 76-year-old retired head teacher. Insomnia had been a problem for decades, yet she had never thought to seek help for it until she heard of a relative's experience. In therapy, she was asked in the assessment session if she had ever experienced any traumas in her life. She sincerely believed there had been none worth a second glance, and said so. In the second session, however, she casually mentioned a lifetime of nightmares of 'cataclysmic awfulness', and recalled she had experienced one only the previous day. 'I woke up, trembling in the dark and thought I was going to die,' she said. 'There's something terrifying about the dark, but it isn't just that. The dreams are about menace, danger.'

The therapist said, 'What is sleep but being in the dark? Somehow you must have linked the two in your unconscious mind and this is where the distress is flooding in. Are you sure there were no traumas in your life?' Then, as if nudged into awareness at last through that gentle enquiry, Sarah spoke diffidently about an incident that happened when she was seven. Diffident, because she was at pains to make it sound as if the horror was not all that profound – after all, it was only a game gone wrong.

" I was at a children's party in a big old house and someone suggested we all go out to play in the garden. There was a small tower in the corner, and some older boys pushed me inside and pretended to lock the door. More children were pushed in, however, until I found myself at the bottom of a pile of bodies – a bit like the Black Hole of Calcutta! Everyone but me was laughing, trying to be brave perhaps. But when the door was shut, seemingly for the last time, it was pitch dark and I couldn't breathe easily because of the weight of children sprawled on my chest. I remember panicking and feeling trapped, even though we were probably released in minutes.

(personal communication) "

It was not long before Sarah, with her therapist's encouragement, came to understand that the party game had created and laid down terrors deep in her memory, deemed trivial by her conscious mind and relegated to the dark, in both senses. Her insomnia she had explained away to herself as a consequence of the stresses in her responsible job; exhaustion from work would indeed plausibly obscure the symptom while she continued teaching. But when retirement threw the problem into the spotlight, she determined not to have what was left of her life ruined by poor quality sleep.

In therapy, she learned her conscious mind might have been too dismissive to consider the childhood episode important; her unconscious, though blanked off, knew otherwise. As Sarah said, 'My hidden controller seemed bent on frightening me, ruining my life for no reason other than spite. Now I realize the opposite is true. It was desperate to be relieved of its fears, and the nightmares were the only route it could take. Like a wake-up call, it could only use an intense approach. But what a pity I left it until I was in my seventies before I could listen to the real message.'

We have already seen how hidden controllers are usually creating havoc – like any ignored child – because their needs have gone unnoticed. The above cases illustrate this simply enough and are included because of their stark messages. But of course, the dramatis personae we carry in our unconscious minds are infinite in their narratives, the depth and severity of their distresses almost beyond description and more complex to offer here.

But more will be discussed briefly in later chapters, where clients who exhibit, say, schizoid behaviour within their relationship usually have a history of childhood emotional deprivation. Their unconsciously remembered guardedness can block normal interaction, particularly so with their partner when they are under some form of resonating stress, which obviously contributes nothing but further chaos to the relationship. Their cut-off emotional responses, replicating their survival technique when little, baffle and infuriate their mates now. The task then is to convince the elusive, distressed child within that they are being seen and heard at last, and can risk coming out to talk at adult level.

It must be acknowledged at this point that there are members of the inner world cast list who have no identifiable disturbance, disabling neurosis or significant past hurts. Split off in the dark they may be, yet for comparatively innocuous reasons: shyness perhaps, or a profound sensitivity which prefers to remain largely obscured to the external world and prompts the conscious mind – if it can – to safeguard its welfare. We all know of boisterous families where one child seems alien or withdrawn. There may be no clinical reason for this seeming difference from their siblings. The child simply is shy, no trauma lurking behind them. Genes play their part too; an ancestral voice may be speaking quietly in the twenty-first century because great-great-grandmother was shy and timid 150 years ago.

Fear and insecurity usually account for the fragmentation of personality within the 'normal neurotic' band, which could apply as much to ourselves as to those clients who come to our consulting rooms. Beyond agreeing that in an ideal world we should all access whatever drives our hidden controllers – inviting them out and consciously integrating them – at this stage in human evolution we are obliged to rest content by doing what we can, with our limited knowledge, for whom we can. If most of our mind lies under the sea like an iceberg we must be thankful that the early psychological pioneers (Freud, Jung, *et al.*) had the insight they did to guide their followers to this point. Perhaps the foregoing accounts will give a greater sense of the mysterious depths we are all touched by, or possess in ourselves, even though no definitive explanation is yet at our disposal.

CASE STUDY
The hidden ally

Journalist Helen Derek was worried about a lump in her breast she noticed one Friday. Panic-stricken, she decided to try a visualizing technique she had practised a little to ask her unconscious mind for information before she booked an appointment to see her doctor after the weekend. She lay on the floor, breathing as she had been taught, covering her eyes with a scarf. One by one, images filled her mind's eye or inner 'screen', each more baffling than the next, until after waiting another few minutes for some kind of coherent pattern (and failing) she pulled the scarf from her eyes, exasperated. She recalls:

> ❝ I had seen a brown-paper-covered exercise book float in and out of vision, followed by a diagram of a dome-like object with

holes, such as a slice of Emmental cheese might look. Next, a rat appeared in the 'picture' – so with that, I lost patience with the silly exercise and went downstairs. Opening the living room door, the first thing I noticed to my right were the bookshelves, and glimpsed a brown-paper-covered exercise book, tightly wedged between textbooks my stepdaughter had left in storage after she'd qualified as an occupational therapist and gone to work abroad. I had never even glanced at them before, wasn't interested. Yet here was this little book inviting inspection. It was difficult to tease out, but when I did the pages fell open to show a diagramatic section of a human breast, the glandular system and a reference to laboratory research – using *rats* – in which hormone activity explained incidents of benign swelling. I was, of course, dumbfounded at the coincidence; and for the remainder of the weekend felt much calmer. Later medical investigation proved my lump was indeed hormone-induced swelling. I really felt my unconscious mind had been a help. How on earth did some part of me know the contents of this textbook, the page on which the relevant material appeared, why did it fall open there – and why doesn't my hidden ally give other answers to order?

(personal communication) **99**

Many will readily find possible explanations to the first three of Helen's questions, but few would want to tackle the last. It is the sheer unpredictability of our unconscious mind that holds such tantalizing quality. Literary giants, composers, scientists and inventors often report their best work came as a result of a dream, or a daydreaming hunch. A young international chess player once confided to me that he set up a board by his bedside on which a difficult move had been posed, for top chess players across the world. He deliberately pored over the problem – without a solution – before turning out the light. He slept dreamlessly and when he woke he knew at once the winning move he should make.

Analytical psychotherapist Nathan Field remarks in his book *Breakdown and Breakthrough*: 'We are obliged to realize that reality manifests not only at the familiar level of waking consciousness but operates in several other dimensions as well, each carrying its own validity. This has a crucial bearing on our understanding of consciousness in general and on psychotherapy in particular' (1996: 37). Field goes on to suggest that we have to grapple with the mystery of how a thought, feeling, fantasy, even an entire personality, can be projected from one psyche into another because we are operating with an inadequate model of the mind:

> 66 We are faced with the whole problem of transmission only because we assume that the parties involved are separate entities to begin with. But if, at some unconscious level, *they are already merged* no transfer is required, since in a state of merger what happens to one happens to the other. Given the fact that each of us feels ourself to be, and looks to others to be, a separate individual, the notion that we also exist in a state of merger puts a heavy strain on our credulity. We can allow the poet licence to declare that 'no man is an island', but to accept it as a literal truth is a different matter. But this, in fact, was Jung's position. He compared individual consciousness to islands standing up in the sea; if we look below the surface we realize that at the level of the seabed we are joined. Somehow we have to entertain the paradoxical notion that, as living beings, we are both separate and united.
>
> (1996: 42) 99

The analogy of our unconscious states being likened to the hidden iceberg (or Jung's islands) and Field's notion that at the level of the seabed we are joined is, of course, both apt and complementary. It gives meaning in my view to the idea that ally and demon can and do co-exist, the latter gravely misunderstood: witness Leo's initial conviction that a demon was controlling his life with malicious intent. It might also explain why the teenage chess player could rejoice in having an ally on tap, ready to deliver solutions to difficult problems overnight. In the sleep state he was free to dive down to the seabed, somehow knowing how and where to find those solutions. It is a fascinating concept.

Others claim to be able to achieve similar connections by meditating, monks being an obvious example. The Venerable Matthieu Ricard, author of *The Art of Meditation* (2010), said in an interview with Jake Wallis Simons for *The Times*: 'The mind trumps all. If you have inner peace, then whatever happens, you are going to be fine' (2010: 9). This philosophy is one cherished by arts teacher Alan Jones (not his real name) whose quiet meditative private life served him well to endure the sorrow when his wife's Alzheimer illness prevented Hilary from speaking anything but incoherent babble. For nearly a year, hospitalized because she was no longer capable of standing or controlling her body, all the communication the couple could consciously enjoy lay in holding hands, Hilary sometimes squeezing his as if in some understanding. Then one evening, on his second visit of the day to kiss her goodnight, suddenly Hilary said clearly, 'Mother dying.' Alan's first thought was that as a loving mother and grandmother to her big family, Hilary was temporarily able to formulate two words to convey she understood she had reached the end of her life.

When at breakfast time next day the telephone rang, he faced the painful possibility of hearing sad news from the hospital. But it was his sister-in-law ringing from the south of France to tell him that the sisters' elderly mother had died overnight. How could Hilary – unable to speak for nine months – clearly announce the fact of an event while it was happening, when no one in the family (including Alan) had any idea the robust old lady was on the brink of death? Could this be yet another clue to add substance to the premise that at some level our unconscious minds merge, that we know much more than we think we do?

CASE STUDY
Long-distance meeting

Before we leave the topic of unconscious communication (at least for the time being, because it is a central theme to support this book's rationale in the context of much of relationship therapy) we should consider Louise. She was a client who presented with grief issues following the death of her husband two years earlier. Childless, she felt all alone and greatly in need of warmth and affection. One winter's night, she dreamed of meeting an old colleague with whom she had lost touch nearly 40 years earlier. In the dream, she was standing on high ground overlooking boats sailing across a bay in high summer. Her old friend appeared with dusty rubble on his hands, explaining his photographic studio had caught fire. The capital letter 'A' seemed written across the scene.

Next day, my client telephoned their former workplace. 'Any idea where John went?' The response was vague. Was it the United States he had emigrated to, or maybe Australia? Obviously the latter sounded hopeful, but it took several more calls before she spoke to someone who volunteered that John's freelance photography had taken him to retirement in New Zealand. In the end, fortunate because her previous career enabled her to quiz professional agencies, she found out he lived in Auckland. John's name was still listed with directory enquiries and within a few hours she was talking to her old friend.

> 66   He couldn't believe I was calling him, because only the previous day (maybe when I was asleep my side of the globe) he had been thinking of me when he took delivery of a rare car he remembered I once owned when we worked together. And yes, his house overlooked a bay, yes he owned a sailing boat but no, his photographic studio had not caught fire. However, three nights later John called me from Auckland: some equipment in his studio

had fused, then burst into flames and done a lot of structural damage. He had that very day been clearing rubble, so of course there was dust on his hands. How on earth did I see that vivid scene? And how could I have had a prevision of his fire?

(personal communication) **99**

This is a strange story, all the more so because of the indisputable time jump in her narrative, remarkable in itself for the detail and location. It opens up vast areas of further exploration in which linear time has no meaning. As neuroscientist Karl Pribram suggests, the human brain itself functions holographically, constructing our reality by interpreting frequencies from another 'domain' that, like Einstein's fourth dimension, transcends time and space (1982: 27–34).

All we know here is that Louise's unconscious mind (apparently with easy access to this domain) had provided her with a gift: somehow it knew where to find John, that he would welcome seeing her again now that he too was widowed. All his personal life until their telephone call was unknown to my client. Then, within months, they were reunited in person, 40 years after their professional friendship had ended. Today, Louise has warmth and affection in her life, married to John, their grief issues resolved not by psychotherapy but by a dream.

So, what has this got to do with relationship therapy? First, we need to acknowledge that for Louise and John a beneficial link-up really happened, where unrecognized parts of themselves were unaccountably involved in proactive healing. Second, if we accept the fact of the existence of powerful hidden controllers, then we must embrace their significance and wonder how much of our present-day emotional distresses arise because we fail to recognize that the demon might be our guide.

When clients realize that the driving force behind what seems at times negative destructiveness is actually benign in intent, then the healing can start. Field again:

66 Having set out to investigate the riddles posed by phenomena such as transference and projective identification, we are led to what must seem blatantly unscientific speculations. Yet serious support for such ideas has been coming from science itself for many years – from contemporary research in physics, mathematics, astronomy, and the major life sciences. The gathering evidence, for example in mind and brain research, has developed into a field of study that is expanding with unprecedented rapidity.

(1996: 43) **99**

Early terrors

Once clients – adults like Leo and Sarah – appreciate how simply their inner world has held early terrors in a frozen lock, desperate for help, then awareness can take over. The therapist leads them towards reintegration of the split-off parts and in so doing encourages them to feel safer to function exclusively from their grown-up self. (There will be regressions, of course, but once the client is aware of their hidden youthful characters, sparked into action once more perhaps by the unexpected, they can learn to manage the outburst.) It is not so simple, however, for a very young child.

A baby knows unerringly what mother is feeling, both consciously and unconsciously, this being an extension of the umbilical psychic bond (benign or malign) experienced in utero; clearly it is pre-verbal. If an unhappy mother's eyes are unloving, unaffirming of her baby's existence, then the messages which the infant receives are negative and terrifying. As Adam Phillips explains in his book *Winnicott*, not to be seen by the mother, at least at the moment of the spontaneous gesture, is not to exist. He goes on to say:

> In Winnicott's account, being seen by the mother is being recognized for who one is, and what the infant is, is what he feels. The infant cannot risk looking, if looking draws a blank; he must get something of himself back from what he looks at. This makes the mother of infancy the arbiter of the infant's truth. Her responsive recognition – not, for example, a conflict of recognitions between them – makes up his sense of himself. The mother is the constitutive witness of the True Self. If she violates the infant's initial omnipotence – forcing him to see her – she 'insults' the infant's self and drives it into hiding. Everything hinges on the changeover from mother as a subjective object to an object objectively perceived; from seeing himself through the other, to seeing the other.
>
> (2007: 130)

In a previous publication (March-Smith 2005), I refer to Julia who offers an interesting illustration of how long-term, devastating damage was caused unwittingly by her mother, struggling with post-natal psychosis. Julia learned in her infancy that eye contact was frightening, a reflection of dark, menacing depths, 'eyes of death', as Jungian analyst Sylvia Perera tells us from Sumerian mythology: 'Those eyes are pitiless, not personally caring. Such eyes bring psychosis; we see them in individuals suffering psychotic states, where the capacity to see through the tightly held fragment to the life process and spirit, in which the static frame inheres as a partial fact, is lost' (1981: 31).

Depression is almost inevitable for the child who experienced mother's eyes where 'all looks dead'. As a result of her early experience, Julia learned in time to avoid looking at all. So adept did Julia eventually become at avoiding seeing into another's eyes that she appeared to be gazing intently at them whereas in reality focusing on the speaker's upper lip, the tip of their nose or chin. Her husband had never realized she did not know what colour his eyes were. Even her therapist was incredulous (on being told the truth) that for several years the two had conducted their professionally intimate relationship, chair opposite chair, without her appreciating that Julia's large, sympathetic eyes never actually looked into her own, as she believed. I wrote:

> ❝ The price Julia paid for this extraordinary avoidance mechanism was a constant feeling of being removed from the centre of life, a half-deadness that paralleled the deadness in her sick mother's eyes so long ago. Naturally, depression dogged her, suppressing her anger that she had not been welcomed lovingly as a baby, that her presence had been seemingly a source of irritation and grief. In therapy, Julia learned first to look at herself in a mirror; then into her therapist's eyes; then into her husband's and close friends' eyes. It was hard for her, and often she regressed to the habitual pattern. Eventually, she found the 'eyes of life' and of love primarily for herself and finally simply for the joy of living.
> (March-Smith 2005: 53–4) ❞

Psychoanalyst Robert Stolorow, best known for his writing on the intersubjective system perspective, offers that psychological conflict develops when a child's central affect states cannot be integrated because they evoke massive or consistent malattunement from caregivers. In other words, there is a breakdown in the child–caregiver system of regulation:

> ❝ This leads to the child's loss of affect-integrating capacity and thereby to an unbearable, overwhelmed, disorganised state. Painful or frightening affect becomes traumatic when the attunement that the child needs to assist in its tolerance, containment, and integration is profoundly absent. . . . One consequence of development trauma, relationally conceived, is that affect states take on enduring, crushing meanings. From recurring experiences of malattunement, the child acquires the unconscious conviction that unmet developmental yearnings and reactive painful feeling states are manifestations of a loathsome defect or of an inherent inner

badness. . . . Thereafter, the emergence of prohibited affect is experienced as a failure to embody the required ideal – an exposure of the underlying essential defectiveness or badness – and is accompanied by feelings of isolation, shame, and self loathing.

(2007: 3–4) **"**

Developmental trauma will, according to Stolorow, constrict and narrow the horizons of emotional experiencing so as to exclude whatever feels unacceptable, intolerable, or too dangerous. Thus we turn back to Leo, offering some degree of illustration here, anxiously conducting his life with half an eye, as it were, to avoid humiliation because he had been exposed too long to family ridicule. As with Julia, a safe, emotional holding had been the missing element in his childhood home life, where his mother's long-term unpredictable responses confused and bewildered him. This was qualitatively different from Julia's infant trauma, however, receiving as she did no affirming expression throughout her mother's psychotic episode: this evoked more serious splitting off.

Projected dread

When Leo reported being bullied at school, his mother laughed. When he was sent away during a family crisis to an unloved (and unloving) grandmother, giving him the same mean-spirited treatment once meted out to her daughter, his tears were ignored and he was punished for being uncooperative. Small wonder he went into adult life with narrowed horizons of expectation: he shuddered from risk taking, from exploring the world, and led – until his bladder somatized high stress levels – a sheltered if limited existence.

Once the core issue pertaining to his panic attacks and dread of humiliating damp patches at his workplace had been discovered, we had more work to do. Leo wanted to look at his fear of standing up for himself, not only with his peers and managers but in his marriage too. 'I dread a backlash of some sort, but I can never put my finger on *what*, and even when I know that Susan wouldn't deliberately cause me hurt, I am still afraid of her. How pathetic is that?'

Clearly Leo was still struggling with ancient material (how could a vulnerable little boy stand up for himself when his family sniggered at the Peter Pan incident?). His wife Susan was unwittingly on the receiving end of that child's projected dread, herself unable to understand why her partner was acting like a wimp towards her, and at work. But the scenario was not as straightforward as it sounds. That same small boy, though frightened of speaking up for himself and telling his tormentors to stop, had brooded ever since. His fury at their belittling jokes was real enough, but he still lacked a voice, his anger as fresh as ever in his unconscious, where time stands still. What he could allow himself for release, however, was in making snide, wounding remarks to Susan (representing his family now), more sulky than full-blown rage. As his therapy progressed, he was encouraged to let those feelings surface, along with the other memories. We used a Gestalt method to release them: that of speaking to an empty chair, as if addressing the people he wanted to shout at, but had never dared.

'What do you really want to say to your parents?' I asked him. 'Imagine they are there, in front of you in those two chairs. Here is your chance to tell them how hurt they made you feel, how angry you are with them. They won't know a thing about what happens today if you prefer never to speak to them about it in reality.'

Leo flinched at first. Talking to an empty chair can be quite inhibiting. But he haltingly began to describe his pain, the endless rounds of excruciating embarrassment at their thoughtless jibes. 'HOW DARE YOU DO THIS TO ME?' he yelled suddenly to the chairs. 'Do you realize how awful you made me feel? It's not FAIR, and I will never forgive you.'

Sometimes I will quickly go and sit in the vacant chair and take on the role of the absent person: it can help encourage out more rage, by justifying 'oneself' or trying to laugh off yet another misunderstanding. I tried it this time. 'Oh, Leo, your Dad and I were only having a bit of fun – you shouldn't get so upset, it's silly of you. Why can't you be more grown up, like your sister?' At this, the child still smarting inside my adult client, stared at me (playing his mother), looked as if he was witnessing a video recording of scenes in his childhood, and he started to cry. 'You mustn't call me silly. I have a right to get upset. It's wrong to have laughed at me.' Leo let the tears run down his cheeks, at last fully conscious of a broken heart at his parents' betrayal.

We later discussed what had happened that day with the chairs. He had found a voice, expressed his feelings – and there had been no feared backlash. Actually, he said, he felt surprisingly free and buoyant. Did this mean he had put his dread behind him now? Leo agreed to wait and see (there are often residual layers of trauma needing exposure before a client feels safe enough to function only from adult). But the signs were good. He began reporting lively rows at home, where he said just what he felt without holding back. 'Susan didn't like it at first. But I told her she couldn't complain about me being a wimp *and* outspoken! This has given me a sense of empowerment I've never known before. I have a voice in the office, too, and I am amazed how people I feared would ridicule me [more parent projection] have responded positively and fairly to suggestions I've made, or criticisms I felt needed to be offered in the best interests of the workplace. . . . Life is opening up at last.'

CASE STUDY
Remote control

A young supervisee telephoned in a panic. 'I think I'm losing my client, Ruby. She's threatening to leave and I have absolutely no idea why.' Not having my notes to hand, I asked her to sum up in the five minutes we had available the gist of her current concern.

66 When I went abroad for three weeks a few months ago, Ruby asked me for the name of another therapist she might turn to if she needed help on an emergency basis. I gave her three names, and learned later that she had found one of them a 'kind, gentle older woman' who did indeed help. But then I realized Ruby was still seeing her, at the same time as she was seeing me, which I explained to her was not appropriate. It occurred to me from what she had been saying that she was getting an easy ride with the 'kind, older woman', and – like a child – wanted to make me feel guilty I wasn't getting it right in her therapy.

(personal communication) 99

Did Ruby have a history where a grandmother and mother were present in her childhood? 'Oh, yes! Father left home and Ruby was reared by two warring women, Grandma and Mum. She learned fast to set one off against the other, getting as she thought the best of both worlds with rewards and treats. But that gave her no real sense of emotional security, did it?' Indeed not. And, in her panicky five-minute call, my supervisee was demonstrating how she was herself unconsciously picking up the sense of unease which her client's permanent state of insecurity evoked, trying as she did as a child to control her emotional well-being by pitting the two carers against one another. Probably her therapist's foreign travels had triggered the regression, unconsciously reminding Ruby of the responsibility she had felt as a child in keeping both women on her side for emotional survival. This is likely to have made her angry without understanding why: that it should not have been necessary to work so hard for love, her natural birthright. So she began to punish her therapist by threatening to leave.

'Ruby will go off to "Grandma" (the older therapist), complaining about your uncaring treatment of her, or whatever, repeating the old pattern of ding-dong between her original carers,' I suggested. 'It's important for her that you refuse to let this situation continue. She must choose between you and the other, showing her at last that boundaries are a vital component in relation-ships, and that she will learn this better by staying in one alliance without rewards or punishments.'

Here we have a different slant on the same theme: that of powerful hidden control from a split-off or frozen part of the self, behaving this time not in a distressed reactive way (such as Leo and Sarah experienced) but proactively setting up what was familiar and, in its own way, had worked for Ruby as a child. Though unaware of the reason behind her driven behaviour, her intent now – to create warring therapists/carers she imagined she could manipulate so they would compete for her – was to re-enact her unhealthy childhood.

The ally within would have to wait a little longer for the counselling process to turn that patterning round. We should never underestimate the lure of the familiar. In well-documented research, we know that battered children taken away from their destructive parents by social workers for their own safety would – if given the choice – usually prefer to return home rather than meet new situations.

Summary

Our powerful hidden controllers exert extraordinary influence decades after their original needs were forged. Mostly, they operate in a frozen time warp, where a child's view persists as if it were yesterday. Whenever our lives or those of our partners manifest distress or some other intense emotion which makes no sense, it is likely urgent messages have been triggered by some resonance with the past; they emerge from the unconscious realms in need of attention.

Because of the frightening intensity sometimes, these 'messages' appear to be demonic, but when therapy reveals their true purpose, those terrifying or absurd symptoms melt away, as if the job has been completed. We have also seen that, in the world of the 'normal neurotic' (there being no scope here to discuss the vast field of fragmentation in serious mental disorder, about which I am anyway not qualified to write), there appears often to be a benign force behind our crises. It urges towards healing, much as a plant forces its way through dark and often stony, resistant earth.

Our hidden controllers invariably represent a much younger part of the self – from our infancy, childhood or adolescence – damaged or traumatized by lacks and inconsistencies in the distant past, however slight. But the internal cast also includes friendly, helpful parts of the unconscious mind which seem to have an uncanny ability to provide information normally outside the scope of our current understanding.

If we take the view of Jung and many others, however, there is a possibility that we possess psyches that connect with each other, merging at some fathomless level; and that this might account for the incidence of telepathy, prevision, Jung's theories of synchronicity (described in his *Memories, Dreams and Reflections*, 1995, first published in the middle of the last century), and his thoughts on the collective unconscious. It may also explain the creative quality of interaction which can occur spontaneously between counsellor or psychotherapist and client in which those concerned are aware of a powerful synergy in the room.

When working with clients it is important to understand that their presenting problems are likely to prove only the tip of the iceberg: symptoms such as anger or grievance, fear or grief may be merely signposts. We must realize that behind the adult's story there usually lurks a hurt child, and that it is the therapist's task to find out what the core issues are and how to reach that child. The next chapter sets out to address ways in which we might achieve this.

2 The search for core issues

In a world increasingly demanding speedy delivery, the concept of brief therapy has become almost a necessity, however much many may deplore the trend when thorough, long-term work has so long been the ideal. From the integrative perspective it is possible to lean heavily on the classical theories while also breaking the rules: for example, where once non-directiveness was regarded as essential practice, we see far more proactive intervention these days. Carl Rogers's ground-breaking work, developed in his book *On Becoming a Person* (1961), discusses the value of the person-centred approach and rightly earned Rogers the accolade of being a founding father of humanistic psychology.

But holding the view that the client knows the answers, that we have only to wait for them to emerge in the process of months (if not years) of therapy seems out of step with the time constraints we face today. Counsellors in GP practices and counsellors and therapists working for Employee Assistance Programme agencies are all under pressure to achieve some satisfactory conclusion within a limited time frame, lamentably (at the time of writing this) sometimes in as short a period as four to six sessions only.

Even in the private sector, economic constraints weigh heavily; these are facts nobody can ignore. Looking back to the last century, the gently meandering Rogerian approach seems ideal, but by current standards almost luxurious. A young trainee, watching one of Carl Rogers's famed filmed sessions was surprised to hear later that what she took for a second or third session was in fact the twenty-eighth with his client.

In contrast, Gestalt psychotherapist Richard Hycner, author of *Between Person and Person: Toward a Dialogical Psychotherapy* (1993), who specializes in relationship therapy and lectures internationally, told a group of colleagues at a UK seminar in 2009: 'As a couples therapist I have to be incredibly active. I purposely point out things, I'm interruptive and engaging. If I am not, I won't have the impact the couple need to interrupt their negative patterns. It's essential to identify repeating patterns.'

So times have changed. A challenge faces us all to find ever more new ways, hopefully without compromise, to speed the process. It is usually clear in the first hour or two what the core issues are likely to be. But a word of caution here: any practitioner would be foolhardy to make snap assessments and not hold an open mind to what might come next as the sessions continue. As Patrick Casement warns in the introduction to his book *On Learning From The Patient*:

> 66 There is a common myth that the experienced analyst or therapist understands the patient swiftly and unerringly. Although some patients try to oppose this, risking the retort that they are 'resisting', other patients do expect it. Perhaps it satisfies a wish to find certainty. Some therapists also appear to expect it of themselves; perhaps to gratify an unacknowledged wish to be knowledgeable or powerful.
>
> (1985: xi) 99

Nobody could quarrel with Casement's thoughts; the caveat is noted. But we live and work in different times now, where somehow those needs – if needs there be – must be acknowledged and overcome, for the common good. Clients appreciate feedback, such as hearing what early impressions are, even though many therapists in the past would have withheld observations in the interests (as they saw it) of the client's slowly unfolding story; or they might have felt a professional reluctance to risk invasion by making premature interventions. Yet identifying unconscious drives early on is, as we have already seen, often crucial. It is the practitioner's job not only to pinpoint as soon as possible how unconscious clues inform the presenting problem, but to convey in due course to their client where they feel the trouble really lies.

Before moving on to discuss case studies to help illustrate this, perhaps it would be appropriate to draw a distinction here between what is commonly held to be brief therapy and what is meant by the phrase in this book. Identifying the heart of the problem and working with it in as short a time as might be available, whether it is in crisis intervention or longer term private practice, is certainly shared ground. But brief therapy, whose founding proponents include Milton Erikson and Richard Bandler, co-founder of neuro-linguistic programming, holds that it is less important to find out how a problem was created than it is in identifying how present factors sustain it, so blocking change.

As we have seen, pinpointing the long-ago cause of the current problem is central to the thrust of these chapters. In using the term brief therapy, therefore, we may have semantic agreement, but a difference of viewpoint. Valuable work is unequivocally achieved by therapists from all disciplines and in a wide spectrum of timescales. But it is usually the quality of the relationship between therapist and client which has a major bearing on the positivity of outcomes. Length of duration does not necessarily mean a thorough or better job done.

Vital leads still get missed, transference issues accidentally ignored, and the alliance breaks down for inexplicable reasons; this, even after years of therapy.

CASE STUDY

Hunger for closeness

When Betty walked into the room, she thought she had come for some grief work because her husband had walked out of the marriage after 20 years together. Heartbroken, baffled, she sat wringing her hands as she began to talk about their 'happy life'. What were those hands conveying, I wondered – were they imploring, begging for something far removed from the current topic, yet clearly central to her existence? What did she crave, was still hungry for?

After half an hour, she had spoken about many occasions when family anniversaries, holidays, special days, even Sunday lunches were seemingly extra-important for her. She had a constant need for all four of her children (now teenagers) and her husband to enjoy them with her. It was priority, no excuses.

'You place a good deal of emphasis on those family gatherings – it's almost as if your life depends on them honouring every date suggested,' I commented. 'Don't they have other things to do sometimes?' The wringing hands almost intensified their movement as she replied, 'Oh no! We are such a happy family, we love being so close – we always do everything together. That's why it's such a shock Harry has left.'

Yet no surprise he had left. My sense was that Harry stayed as long as he could for the sake of their children, but that Betty's neediness was increasingly a serious blight on their relationship, doubtless cushioned over the earlier years of their marriage by having a young family. Her craving for being in the centre of domestic life, at her most happy building up to and including its heydays, was neurotic. So, the core issue was her hunger for closeness, intimacy – not in the marriage bed so much as in the preparation and execution of family meals. What did this suggest?

The next half hour had Betty describing her childhood, how her railway worker father would arrive home tired out at seven in the evening, taking over responsibility (in reality sleeping in front of the television) from her mother, who had rushed out to work cleaning offices. Their joint income was useful – it paid for family holidays – but Betty agreed weekday evenings (with her little sister asleep in bed) were lonely and boring. 'But the weekends weren't! I lived for them, because that was when my Mum cooked lovely meals and me and my younger sister helped her dish up the Sunday roast.'

Betty had unconsciously tried to recreate those comforting special days by making her own family sit round the table for every meal; together wherever possible except for school lunchtime and activities. Harry was, of course, encouraged to drop by for a snack on his daily rounds as a plumber. He had no life of his own; nor had she. Finally, Harry found the courage to wrench himself free from such relentless demands.

Ask a neighbour before his departure, and they would have described next door's family as devoted. Ask Betty and she would nod approval at their perception. Ask Harry and the teenagers and their response would almost certainly be different. Yet Betty presented herself for therapy because she wanted help to overcome grief and anger, to learn how to live without her husband. She was completely unaware of the pivotal role her childhood frustrations had played in the breakdown of their marriage. As the therapy session swiftly moved on to talking about this, Betty's wringing hands slowly calmed down. They even, at some point of recognition, spread outwards as if in acceptance. Once, she smiled and acknowledged, 'Yes, I put my hand up to that . . . I did expect too much attention from Harry.'

The severity of her task in coming to terms with the collapse of her marriage would now be considerably lessened, thanks to her insight. Once her hidden controller (in this case, her emotionally starved little girl) had been identified in session, owned and accepted, Betty began to see her adult life as hugely influenced by that little girl's conviction that happiness lay in cosy togetherness. Her belief effectively produced the opposite: the misery of abandonment. Chastened by the revelations, Betty nonetheless realized what lay behind her 'family feeding frenzies', and this alone gave her enough understanding to monitor her behaviour carefully in the future.

No one could claim this was a case of serious childhood deprivation. There was no abuse involved, no cruelty, no trauma. Betty's parents did what they thought was right by working hard in the interests of bringing enough money into the home to give their children occasional treats and memorable family holidays. It is an attitude found in many households these days, where two incomes are essential to pay the mortgage or keep the rent paid. Yet Betty clearly suffered as a little girl, demonstrably so because she and her own family were affected by its legacy. Another set of parents might have taken more care to make the children feel emotionally nourished during the week: more cuddles, lively interest in their friendships and schoolwork, giving them undivided attention when they needed it. The point here is that a humdrum upbringing, whom nobody could challenge as actually wrong, still produced a significant neurosis in the next generation.

When the great Russian composer Tchaikovsky was a little boy, his parents took their apprehensive son in a horse-drawn carriage to his first boarding school. As the carriage moved off again, we are told by Christopher Nupen in his Channel 4 television documentary (2009) that the boy clung to the wheels weeping hysterically as he tried to stop their departure. I know of a modern schoolboy who, dropped at the gates of his new boarding school, clung in similar fashion to his parents' car, desperately grabbing at the door handle and only letting go when the car slowly gathered speed (and his father realized what was happening).

Both boys' anxiety at separation from their mothers on those two historically different periods are the same anxieties felt by countless children when they face abandonment, real or imagined. Their memories linger in their unconscious world and influence adult relationships: broken trust, a sense of betrayal, a hardening against further hurt – all this and more often lie behind a client's current presenting problem.

Inexplicable absences of one or other parent for hospital visits or, as sick patients themselves, children suddenly finding they were alone among strangers, some of whom would medically have been forced to cause them pain – these terrifying experiences are reported time and again. Middle-aged men and women shed tears once more as the memories resurface and they recount the horrors they endured when they felt isolated and unloved, perhaps because their hospital in less enlightened times did not allow visits, or travelling difficulties and family constraints made it impossible for parents to come. Gazing through hospital windows (or their sick-bed windows at home) also figures largely in their memories of childhood grief. Although they may not have connected this with their defensive behaviour in current relationships, when encouraged to let them surface fully the client begins to realize how much their fear of further abandonment, or other perceived cavalier treatment on the part of the carer, is controlling them and their interaction with their partner.

Abused children

So far, we have looked at psychological trauma in childhood of comparatively mild severity which nonetheless seeps into adult ways of being. That seepage has had a toxic affect on relationships, as we have already seen in what are straightforward case histories when we consider Leo, Betty and others. If the trauma should be injurious beyond the bewildering hurt described above, we might then ask the question: how much greater the impact on the child? Do wounds score more deeply if a young person has been sexually or physically abused? Does this mean we are entering a different arena altogether? As Gabarino and Gilliam in their book *Understanding Abusive Families* point out: 'Child abuse is not simply less than optimal child rearing. It is a pattern of behaviour that drastically violates both moral and scientific norms concerning child care' (1980: 70–1).

Moira Walker, in her seminal book *Surviving Secrets* warns us: 'It is essential to recognize and acknowledge that abuse of a child leads to huge developmental damage which has ongoing implications. The effects do not simply disappear or evaporate as the child reaches adulthood.' On the same page, Walker writes that children who have been abused do not have high expectations of others, that they do not expect help: 'They often do not have a sense of indignation when they are ill-treated. They do not feel or impart positive messages about themselves. They cannot easily be self-protective' (1992: 1).

This lack of indignation at their abusive treatment, a passive resignation, has a familiar resonance with many of the cases of abuse which come to the attention of therapists and counsellors during the course of their work. Yet a senior NSPCC children's officer once told me that the worst kind of cruelty he had ever encountered was of a small boy (believed by the man of the house to be fathered by his wife's lover) being excluded from all family occasions. The family ate their meals in one room, but the boy was given his to eat in the kitchen, with no explanation. There was no physical abuse, no starvation or neglect and no sexual abuse. But the officer put the emotional torture experienced by this excluded child, allowed to mix with his brothers and sisters but not to eat with them, on a par with criminal deprivation. Once again, we have abandonment and betrayal at the heart of the trauma. What is the likely outcome for this boy? In *Joy. Expanding Awareness* Will Schutz states:

> 66 A person who has too little inclusion, who will be called undersocial, tends to be introverted and withdrawn. Consciously, he wants to maintain this distance between himself and others, and insists that he doesn't want to get enmeshed with people and lose his privacy. But unconsciously, he definitely wants others to pay attention to him. His biggest fears are that people will ignore him, generally have no interest in him, and would just as soon leave him behind. . . . His deepest anxiety, that referring to the self-concept, is that he is worthless.
>
> (1967: 135–6) 99

The emotional wasteland this boy experienced was bound to affect deeply his adult relationships. We can only guess at the fallout, how it would leave him struggling with a pitiable sense of worthlessness, his unloveable self too unacceptable to be allowed to share in that most intimate of family ritual, eating together (Betty's story comes to mind here).

Who can say definitively that the suffering is less or more than that of an eight-year-old girl whose elder brother regularly sexually abused her – described by him as a 'game' – and who kept their secret because she believed revelation would somehow break up the family? Again we see the dread of exclusion, coupled with its potent mix of the lure of the familiar: routine abuse was all she knew (and had become used to), and the family status quo to her was paramount. So she said nothing.

We might ask ourselves here what part the ally in the unconscious – the hidden controller – can play in these terrible accounts. At the risk of sounding simplistic, I would offer that during childhood the ally serves to keep the traumatic memories hidden, or denied, for this is often the means of surviving abuse at our most vulnerable. Moreover, from wide research we know that truly appalling histories can result in profound splitting off, as in psychological fragmentation, fleeing from reality. Walker states:

> The development of Multiple Personality Disorder is an extreme response to equally extreme multiple abuse. . . . Denial is, of course, endemic in abuse. The very nature of denial is that it is not open either to reasoned argument or to accepting evidence: denial is often a successful means of transcending sensible debate. In cases of abuse, there is a constant challenge to reason, since we would prefer to think of some of the facts of abuse as being impossible. This is even more so with multiple personality. Since it occurs in situations where abuse is almost unbelievable in its variety of horrors, the denial of the phenomenon of multiple personality could be interpreted as a denial of these horrors.
> (1992: 113)

Violence and guns

Darla Franey is a counsellor in Oakland, California, specializing in grief and loss in children. Her clientele is largely African American, most youngsters reporting witnessing a member of their family or close friends being killed, usually in street shootings. Oakland has the fourth highest murder rate in all US cities and also a higher than average rate of students who report gang membership. The area has issues with drug dealing, use and abuse, and two-parent homes where children grow up against a low socioeconomic background. These kids need therapy more than most, she reasoned, taking the internship job offered at the city's Circle of Care centre, despite initially fearing for her own safety. Her young clients were referred to her suffering from nightmares, sleeping problems, clingy or aggressive behaviour. The core issues were obvious: but how to reach these children? She told me:

> I use a sand tray a lot. The children choose from a variety of toy figures – people, animals, mythical characters – placing them in key positions on the sand as they tell a story. As the weeks go by, the original 'picture' of the story's theme begins to change as

our work develops. I was seeing a sixth grader (a very aggressive 11-year-old boy who learned to knit as an anxiety-binding activity) who found the sand and toys so compelling he created an epic struggle of good guys versus bad guys. He used dragons, eagles, owls and other animals, with the fight going on for a lot of the session. I made occasional comments, narrating the action, or paraphrasing the things he said until the end, when after this great struggle, the good guys finally defeated the bad.

Picking up the theme of good winning over bad, I was beginning to comment upon this as we were clearing up, when he looked at me with what I now interpret as surprise at my naivety, and said, 'That's a story for little kids, but life really isn't like that.' It was sad that kids this young already know that life isn't always fair, and that good doesn't always win over evil. But this gave us a good starting point, and I believe the work helped him.

(personal communication) **99**

Violence and gang warfare is now endemic on both sides of the Atlantic, as are the continuing tragic cases coming to our attention of drug-fuelled cruelty to children, of terrible neglect, starvation, even murder. We do not need (nor is it appropriate) to discuss here the problems facing social services, mental health workers, the entire field of therapeutic care which is likely to be encountered increasingly in the twenty-first century. We do need to recognize, however, that whichever way we look we are dealing with abuse.

Abuse to the psyche, the body, the spirit of a child – all is damaging, all traumatic for life. The best any therapist or counsellor can hope to achieve is to free some of the burden from the shoulders of these wounded people, much as Darla Franey moved in to help forge still stronger acceptance in her young African American client. Together, over the weeks, they reached understanding: life can be hard, but it need not be lonely. Incredibly, this boy had not split off into multiple personality disorder, despite the violence and loss to which he had been exposed. Somehow, his internal ally had encouraged him forward to reach out to a white woman who visited his school with a sand tray. They made a relationship, she saw into his hell and they shared insight into his suffering. Slowly his story unfolded, with the animals' position and fate giving the counsellor the clues she needed to reach – and heal a little – his core distress.

Now we return to the case of the girl whose abusing brother visited her bedroom once a week. Here we see her hidden ally at work, screening off from her rational mind in those years the inappropriateness of the visits. But when she reached adulthood and a marriage crisis steered her towards counselling that same ally encouraged out the hidden material, at first (as we have seen before) seeming demonic in intent, with panic attacks, nightmares and hysterical distrust of her husband. But a better emotional life was to come.

A matter of timing

Healing is so often a matter of timing. She was ready to be helped to face the unfaceable; her current relationship difficulty could wait. She found herself talking about her early experiences to a woman counsellor, who pointed out her innocence in all of them, how she was bullied by her older brother to perform acts for his pleasure; how emotionally absent her mother must have been, failing to notice all was not as it should have been upstairs. The sessions were not brief. There was far too much work to do over many months integrating this new viewpoint with her current breakdown in relationship with her husband. Small wonder she had presented for counselling for marital guidance. She had no idea her childhood secret had any relevance to the issues of trust which had inevitably emerged with her partner. The past was not all in the past, as many would have it; her distress in the here and now directly linked with childhood betrayal.

The counsellor quickly recognized signs of the probability of past sexual abuse: in the self-effacing manner her client walked into the room, sat with her knees firmly closed together and arms folded, wore a defensive expression and was reluctant to meet her eyes; and as time went on skilfully provided a safe emotional containment, slowly becoming the caring, observant 'mother' the client had lacked. Eventually, healing anger surfaced and the work of integration could begin.

Before we leave the subject of abuse, it might be relevant here to add that it comes in many guises, not always recognizable as such. If the most horrific cases are the dramatic kind – physical, sexual, psychological (as in the excluded boy at mealtimes) – then less obvious situations need our scrutiny too. An over-indulged child, permitted excesses of all kinds to serve a parent's own needs, or a child whose parents have no emotional boundaries, can be said to be the victims of abuse. Wherever lines are broken to provide for another's selfish, neurotic or unstable requirements, we see a vulnerable young person's rights being violated. Subtle rather than gross, the abuse is nonetheless damaging.

A case comes to mind, where a single mother had willingly permitted her daughter to share her bed right up into her teens, only too glad to have her warmth and mutually serving security. Although there was no question of sexual invasion, there was abuse of another kind in that the woman also allowed the little girl to order her about, acting on infantile whims while she experimented with how far she could go. Years later, her daughter had difficulty leaving home, afraid to stand alone without her co-dependent parent on hand to help her face the world outside.

The mother failed to prepare her daughter for independence, driven unconsciously by the need to ensure her daughter's attachment and everlasting love. The hidden controller in this case was the split-off young part of herself who sought to recreate the unhealthy attachment she herself had once experienced with her own mother, perpetuating the cycle. So she had unwittingly betrayed her own child by failing to help her learn autonomy, to discover the values of boundary setting: how far could the little girl push before hearing a firm 'no', for example. It was the mother who presented years later for psychotherapy, in torment as to why her daughter's relationships with men always seemed to go wrong, and why she had turned to drugs in her late twenties.

Over-strict parental control can be equally harmful to a youngster's sense of self. As can irrational demands, pleading neediness, inappropriate expectations of performance or devotion: all affect a growing child's well-being and security. A youngster cannot know what is going on, only that they are not relaxed and at peace with their childhood. They develop a wariness, ever watchful over gauging prevailing moods in the household. The harm lies in their gradual loss of self derived from the psychological vampiring which goes on in dysfunctional homes; vampiring here means to invade the sensitivities of the little person involved, a disregard of his or her own needs and a draining overall of life's emotional blood.

Such abuse leaves its own character of scars. We see them in the consulting room with clients significantly showing high degrees of anxiety, a need to comply and a lack of autonomy; or its opposite, in a subtle show of arrogant defendedness, where the client seeks constantly to volley the ball back across the net as it were, bent on conceding nothing. This is heavy work for the therapist. But if a practitioner, with no emotional investment, finds their extreme guardedness frustrating, consider how their partner might cope in a relationship blighted by such determined resistance? In the next chapter we will look at a few case studies which underline the point.

Before this, we should take a brief look at a few of the theories in the therapist's toolkit, those which owe much to the early pioneers' inspired work in mental health even though time has modified them, as we would expect after a century. There are countless books out there, expertly defining the various schools of thought, from the Freudian approach to latter day solution-based concepts in counselling and psychotherapy. This book is not the place to lay them all out to study. Reference will be made from time to time to key theories on which I base my work, which inform the therapeutic search for core issues in relationship breakdown. Some understanding of them at this juncture may help clarify later discussion.

Background knowledge

As John Rowan says in *The Reality Game: A Guide to Humanistic Counselling and Therapy*, one of the key differences between psychoanalysis and humanistic psychotherapy concerns the concept of **transference:**

> 66 Psychoanalysts regard transference as the single most important element in any therapy which goes deep enough to change the whole character structure. Humanistic psychotherapy and psychoanalysis share the aim of changing character structure, but differ on method – psychoanalysts deny that any method other than transference can go deep enough to achieve this goal. What is transference? Transference is the inappropriate repetition in the present of a relationship [that] was important in a person's early development. . . . The most common form it takes is of the client having strongly positive – perhaps erotic – feelings towards the therapist, or else strongly negative feelings . . . in transference the therapist quite often turns into a loved, hated or feared parent. The client then reacts to that projection rather than to the therapist as a real person.
>
> (1983: 99) 99

Rowan goes on to point out (as we have already learned) that part of our reaction to many events in our lives is under our conscious control, *and part of it comes from unconscious forces* (my italics). We all have these echo chambers in our minds, so that certain words, gestures or actions with the right 'vibration frequency' have the power to evoke a powerful noise in us: 'The therapy situation merely brings this to our attention more, makes it harder to avoid or deny. . . . Transference is there, whether we like it or not, and whether we know it or not. The only question is, what are we going to do with it?' (1983: 100).

Clients apologizing for weeping in the consulting room, showing anxiety about being a little late or early, saying sorry for needing a glass of water or to go to the lavatory, these small illustrations indirectly speak of their transferring, or **projecting** their old fear of authority on to the therapist, of perceiving they are getting it wrong or somehow inconveniencing, annoying the other person.

In the **countertransference** (what the therapist is feeling) I may want to point out gently that they have no need to worry about my reactions (here the Good Mother has been 'called out', aware of wanting to put the frightened child more at ease); but I would usually resist this urge. Yet it can prove quite productive, particularly if I wait for an appropriate segment in that or a later session to illustrate what we are really experiencing together. As in classical analysis, the healing place lies in the neurosis coming out in the room via the quality of the relationship between client and therapist, be it negative, positive – in that order – or in reverse.

When as a trainee I first started working with clients, my new supervisor shamed me into realizing I had betrayed a departing client (after what I thought were two good years together) failing to let her move into (and do battle with) the **negative transference**. The betrayal lay in keeping the positive stuff comfortable for both of us; she professed herself happy with her time with me, work complete. But it was not. We had both dodged confronting her murderous rage at childhood neglect – and I alone was to blame for not realizing we were avoiding it. True, she left more confident, aware of how her adaptive defences were no longer helpful, but the darkly spiteful rage at her mother had not been fully cleared. That rage would inevitably spurt out in some future relationship, the stuff of so many marital breakdowns. Jungian analyst Robert Stein describes the negative transference like this:

> 66 The emotional frustration and disillusionment which the child experienced in the relationship to the parent is reconstellated in the negative transference. This aspect of the analytical relationship must be resolved satisfactorily; if it isn't, the internal union between the masculine and feminine opposites does not occur. This experience is an essential step in the process of re-establishing a connection with one's soul.
>
> (1973: 149) 99

This is a Jungian concept in which archetypes play key roles. In lay terms, we could say that I failed my client all those years ago because I did not enable her to claim her inner protective Father archetype for back-up to release her rage at her primary caregiver. Like her actual father, I also opted out, preferring to keep life sweet in the consulting room by colluding with the status quo, too inexperienced to appreciate what I was failing to provide.

She needed to find a masculine strength in me to help restore balance in her fragmented inner world, where lack of male–female harmony, or soul connection, in her parents' relationship was continuing to play itself out through their daughter's own unhappiness. Like my client, I too had had an ineffectual father who pacified rather than challenged my mother. Only years later, after personal therapy had done its job, could I understand my omission.

A shock for partners

The effect of negative transference on to a counsellor or therapist in session may seem uncomfortable at times, for nobody enjoys being verbally attacked and glared at with hatred, even though a practitioner knows it is projected rage, seldom personal. But now imagine the effect of negative transference on to a partner at home, completely unaware of what is really going on: this onslaught can be emotionally crucifying.

Some hidden controller in the unconscious mind (as we know, a distressed younger part of the self) roars out its pain from earlier trauma, hurling baffling or spiteful remarks which will leave the listener reeling with shock. It had only needed a trigger or resonance (as Rowan has pointed out in the context of the therapeutic relationship) to release black fury. When pain erupts to the surface at last, partners, children, work colleagues, friends could all come into line for the fallout, but partners are by far the most likely to be involved. They after all are the current caretakers, mother or father from another time who will not look the same yet something about their mannerism, vocabulary, facial expression will suddenly spring them to life – it is as if they are now in the room.

The subject of **boundaries** has already been touched upon when we looked at the lack of them having had serious long-term impact on the young girl who was drawn into an unhealthy co-dependent relationship with her mother. It is a topic we find woven into other kinds of family dysfunction, where people do not realize the need to keep boundaries (the brother invading his sister's bedroom being an obvious example) and we will come upon more later. Insensitive parenting where a child's development might have been delayed or distorted with unresolved **Oedipal** issues is likely to be hampered also by failure to understand the need for boundaries in a family triad. Dismissed by many these days as baseless, outdated theory, nonetheless the Oedipus complex as defined by Sigmund Freud (1899), does have, in my view, continuing relevance in the present century.

To conclude this chapter on the search for core issues in trying to ensure a successful outcome to therapy, here are a few other suggestions to encourage that quest. Dreams, however trivial and deemed unimportant by the client, are important signposts or guides to the unconscious world, full of allies (and demons) intent on providing clues to help the healing process. We can learn about interpreting dreams at Jungian workshops or seminars, or from our own personal therapy.

Dreams about animals, however frightening, often represent the ally that longs to convey messages from the shadowy inner world. It is our instinctual self, sometimes urging us to harness more courage, perhaps to 'growl' and stand our ground more often, instead of being too compliant or accommodating, for fear of reprisal. In some tribes it is said it used to be the custom to celebrate terrifying nightmares next day round the camp fire, when the dreamer would be helped to realize that the dream tiger was merely trying to encourage instinct, not destroy.

Archetypal characters (for example, the Wise Old Crone or Wise Old Man) will make their appearance to point the way forward, even though they may appear as ordinary folk in the dream narrative, going about ordinary business: the trick is to see through the haphazard storyline and ask ourselves 'What's really being said here?'

Revealing material

Drawings, such as depicting 'Myself Aged Five', to execute at home in a quiet 15 minutes for discussion at the next session, provide revealing material for the therapist. I was amazed at my own sketch once drawn unaware at a professional workshop. It showed my mother as a huge tree inside the garden gate with branches outstretched in supplication, and the central trunk's rough bark showing a wide open 'mouth', as if begging for emotional nourishment. I had placed myself well out of reach, playing on the road. That sketch said a great deal about the inappropriate role reversal I had found myself having to play, for various family reasons.

Finally, fairy stories can be useful. *The Ugly Duckling* and *Babes in the Wood* have twenty-first century parallels in the therapy room. What practitioner has not witnessed the eventual emergence of a fine swan, no longer trapped in his or her unsympathetic setting in life, or recognized a lost young couple in a forest of confusion, with no belief in a safe way out? Fairy tales are timeless. They reflect the psychic scene, no matter the actual setting. Adult women who still retain a childlike expression, have inappropriate hairstyles and clothes for their age group, frequently lead their life, as it were, under the mantle of the fairy story with which they most identify. There are any number of Rapunzels out there, Snow Whites and Cinderellas, all still looking for their handsome prince (alias father) to rescue them. Asking new clients to name their favourite fairy tale can often help the therapist more clearly to pinpoint a core emotional issue.

This was well illustrated by the arrival of a depressed woman, whose childhood had been deprived both emotionally and financially when her parents separated after bitter rows over money. Hoping not to jar her with such an unexpected question, I casually invited her to tell me the character in a fairy tale with whom she most resonated. Unhesitatingly, came the swift response: '*The Little Match Girl*' (Hans Christian Andersen's short story published in 1845 about a girl dying of cold but afraid to go home penniless because she had sold no matches, lighting them for comfort, one by one). This woman's lifelong search for emotional warmth, and desperate last attempts to create it in a cold marriage, had finally seemed too futile, all hope gone, with suicide into oblivion a tempting conclusion to end it all.

But she had one last 'match' to light: she came into therapy. We could talk then about the little matchstick seller locked away inside her unconscious, too sad to wield any power or challenge her relationship. That would change, in time. Her ally nudged her towards kindling some fire, anger no longer lifeless and turning in on itself but flaring up to produce a fine conflagration of rage in the therapy room.

Depression is often the result of suppressed rage, where childhood taught that ugly demonstrations of negative feelings were dangerous, if not pointless. Healthy responses to early frustration were therefore pushed into the depths of the unconscious, where a little girl or boy deems them too unsafe to unleash again. There they fester, sometimes for decades, sometimes for life, if nothing is done about them. For this woman, after decades of compliance, bound by convention (and, interestingly, concern about coping on her own financially if she should leave the marriage) her desperation finally pushed her towards change.

Summary

Holding an open mind to what might come next is priority for the practitioner, but nonetheless it should be clear in the first few sessions what the core issues are likely to be. What the client presents for the therapist or counsellor to address is sometimes a far cry from that which is really at the centre of their current problem. This is not the result of obfuscation on the client's part: they have no idea what lies at the heart of the distress they feel. This could be long-suppressed ancient material from an unhappy past, or the spillover from their partner's own childhood wounds, or a combination of both. Often a crisis of some sort will bring one or two people into the therapy room, the 'last straw that breaks the camel's back' which forces the pace to try to mend the collapsing relationship.

Abuse comes in many guises, not always of a brutal physical or sexual nature. In working with clients where abuse is suspected, it is important to build up a safe emotional containment within the therapeutic alliance before moving in to talk about the acts of abuse or, indeed, make any allusion to it. Victims are still vulnerable. They need time to wait to sense if they can trust the therapist or counsellor with their secrets. Fear of exclusion (by their family originally, but this flows on into wider areas of contact in adulthood) is usually a powerful reason to keep silent when they are young; also guilt (they may have liked the attention) or feelings of worthlessness soon merge into their conscious mind and they may begin to believe they were somehow to blame.

Sexual abuse leaves a tragic legacy should the secrets perpetuate; the effect on a marriage is often catastrophic if the partner either does not know, or will not accept the situation once told. Therapy's chief objective must be to help the client or clients to understand that the victim was blameless, the lack of safety in their home was not their responsibility, and that betrayal by the perpetrator, or caregiver who failed to check the abuse, was profoundly wounding.

Psychological abuse ranks comparably as damaging as physical or sexual abuse; emotional pain alone can torture a child. In another category again, although not obviously abusive, many practices going on can result in lasting harm to a child. They may be over-indulged to serve a parent's own needs, be required to nourish a parent in a role reversal, or they may have a collusive parent who invades their boundaries inappropriately, similarly to serve their own needs. These youngsters will go out into the world unprepared for the hostile reception their customary behaviour will create. Future relationships will almost certainly suffer.

In order to pinpoint core issues, we need to be acquainted with the classical theories in psychotherapy, as well as the more modern variations expounded in humanistic psychology, Gestalt methodology, intersubjective and attachment theories, and so on; not easily referenced here because of their sheer number and diversity, but readily accessible on the internet or on library shelves. Some understanding of Jungian dream interpretation can be helpful in the therapeutic bond, as is the use of spontaneous drawing and finding out which of the fairy stories in our culture most resonate with the client.

Observing body language is instructive. Notice particular areas of the client's body (the position of hands, legs and arms, and whether they seem comfortable, or otherwise, with face-to-face eye contact), for these will hold clues to internal turmoil. Equally important would be to pay attention to the client's breathing: what is happening? Rapid, shallow movement will suggest, of course, high levels of anxiety; but sometimes that anxiety can reach a point where it is as if they have stopped breathing. It may even be necessary to urge 'Breathe!' Then gently suggest they take a few deep breaths – fill the stomach out first, then take the air up slowly into their lungs – to help calm and ground them, holding the breath for a moment before slowly breathing out. Repeat this exercise half a dozen times until the tension eases. Suggest they practise this at home, ideally stretched out on the floor with their head resting on a book or cushion.

In the next chapter, we meet more of the dramatis personae from the inner world, additional characters inhabiting the unconscious who are forged in childhood to complement and support the frontline defenders.

3   Subpersonalities and their defensive role

The betrayed theatrical clown who cries his despair in the dressing room before having to go on with the show; the famous entertainer who ends his or her life in a reclusive, untimely death – we all recognize this tragic character. They have an archetypal quality, perhaps captured best in our imagination in Leoncavallo's nineteenth-century opera *Pagliacci*, when the clown Canio paints his face for the laughing crowds out there, while weeping in anguish at the loss of his beloved. We see the archetype too in many popular media entertainers over the years, who seem to lead such lonely, eccentric lives. These men and women stir our pity: how is it they can be so funny and successful and yet have been so utterly miserable? The paradox might be better understood if we return to the realm of the inner world.

CASE STUDY

The Comedian or Jester

A client once tried to charm his way into making me laugh, clearly an automatic survival mechanism. Soon it became more obvious that this was his practised way of ensuring safety in a relationship. His performance – spontaneously witty remarks, velvety chuckles – was polished, and not a little seductive. I was beginning to form a picture of a small boy, constantly on the look out to make his mother smile. Why? What was at stake here that made a grown man continue to act out his defensive role in childhood? The answer soon came: the wounds were too profound to change his boyish ways. He still believed he must entertain his mother, here in the consulting room.

    Max was an only child, born a few months after his father had walked out. His mother fell into depression at the abandonment and may (though this was not known) have sunk even further into grief with post-natal mental illness. 'She was *always* in tears,' he recalled. Small wonder her little boy, as soon as he could walk and talk used his antics to try to amuse her in a child's desperate attempt to claim attention.

Now, 50 years later, Max was still driven by his need to win affection. If we compare Julia's history with her mother, we have a clinically interesting difference in the outcome, in that she (who had failed to find validation in her mother's non-seeing eyes, eyes of death as in the Sumerian myth) had grown up afraid to look into anyone's eyes for fear of discovering her 'nothingness' once more, an absent reflection.

Max, on the other hand, must have been initially much more closely bonded with his mother. However despairing, she looked at her new baby with enough visual connection to forge good feeling between the two of them. His comic antics in later years of childhood came from a premature lunge at caregiving, nurturing his mother intuitively to cheer her up so that he might in turn be nurtured.

Ready to end it

Predictably, Max became a doctor, a depressed doctor. The lure of the familiar had steered him towards giving yet more service, working with sick people, and far from fulfilling his life he was ready to end it. His Comedian, or Jester subpersonality, had at last nearly exhausted itself. He was no longer ready to make people laugh to create warmth in the room. When he tried this with me, it felt like the last dregs from his reservoir of seductive charm. Challenged, at first he looked crestfallen, as if his tools of survival were being threatened. In time, he learned to use his considerable gifts only when he wanted to make a joke he could enjoy along with others, to be aware of monitoring his impulse to entertain and, most importantly, to permit himself the luxury of tears instead of blocking them to attend to his mother's grief.

In body language terms, Max was a textbook illustration of Lowen's masochistic character structure, described in his book *Bioenergetics*. As masochism is equated in the public mind with the wish to suffer, or having a perverted need to experience physical pain so that he can enjoy sex, we need to appreciate here that in bioenergetic terms this view is far removed from that assumption. As Lowen explains:

 He does suffer, and since he is unable to change the situation, it is inferred that he wishes to remain in that condition. . . . The masochistic character structure describes an individual who suffers and whines or complains but remains submissive. Submissiveness is the dominant masochistic tendency . . . if [he] shows a submissive attitude in outward behaviour, he is just the opposite inside. On the deeper emotional level, he has strong feelings of spite, negativity, hostility and superiority. However, these feelings are strongly blocked out [for] fear that he would explode in violent behaviour. He counters the fear of exploding by a muscular pattern of holding in. Thick, powerful muscles restrain any direct assertion and allow only the whine or complaint to come through.

(1975: 163) **99**

This is precisely how Max presented: short and thickset, strong musculature round shoulders and buttocks, whining rather than be outspoken at my challenges, yet building up seething resentment internally: his defences had been rumbled and it scared him. Fortunately, as our time together opened up for him a sense of safety in which he could blurt out his negative feelings, we began to build a healthier relationship where he no longer needed to rely upon his seductive wit. He could risk offending his therapist and witness she did not burst into tears. Lowen again:

66 An attitude of submission and pleasing is characteristic of masochistic behaviour. On a conscious level the masochist is identified with trying to please; on the unconscious level, however, this attitude is denied by spite, negativity and hostility. These suppressed feelings must be released before the masochistic individual can respond freely to life situations. . . . The dominant, self-sacrificing mother literally smothers the child, who is made to feel extremely guilty for any attempt to declare his freedom or assert a negative attitude.

(1975: 166) **99**

Max was certainly one such child, totally dependent on his mother for his well-being and totally depended upon for hers. When he left home to study medicine and get married, his choice of bride proved an uncanny replica of the only other woman in his life. His wife suffocated him emotionally, clinging on to their family life together (now with two children), yet with a determined control that had Max once again submissive.

His depression grew in depth as the marital years rolled on. Afraid to alter the status quo, yet fearing any movement outward might prove worse than staying put, he – and his wife – were locked in a stagnant relationship. She too became depressed now that their family had left home. 'I honestly thought one of us would curl up and die, in order to leave our marriage with honour rather than opprobrium,' said Max. And that is what happened; his wife developed a terminal illness and died two years later. Max came into therapy a year after that, about to embark on a new relationship and determined to do what he could to ensure no further repetitions in his life patterning. Aware that his depression started in childhood, he believed he needed help to talk through those early days. He was largely unaware of his seductive defences, his unconscious survival toolkit stacked with disarming charm, of the collusive nature in his marriage where he served another's needs for too long. In due course, he realized quite how much his toddler traumas were still driving his behaviour now.

So where was the powerful hidden controller in this story? As a boy, then later operating in a frozen time warp, Max's belief that he had to keep on entertaining his primary carer (mother, then wife) continued to work for him for as long as he got results: a loving smile, an appreciative chuckle. But his underlying depression, where resentment festered with no release in anger, rebellious outbursts as they should have erupted (particularly in his teens), had finally collapsed into hopelessness.

Where there had been hope as his marriage began, ultimately there was loss of hope. So the controller (his inner small boy) became his demon, each morning silently asking morosely 'What's the point? Why bother at all?', switching off the lights for the Comedian in him. An audience was no longer laughing, it was all too much effort. His depression worsened, but in the months leading up to the death of his wife, his Jester/Comedian subpersonality once more rose wearily to the occasion, just in case it would spark new life.

When Max first came into therapy automatically he went through the motions again, trying to win smiling approval from a woman. Yet there was a psychic exhaustion in the room, painful to witness. His ally-cum-demon had brought him – at the crucial, timely point of breakdown – and now there was urgent work to do.

The need to protect

As we have seen, clues to discover the core issues in a client's presenting problem will often lie in identifying their operating subpersonalities. 'Normal neurotic' people tend to have their internal dramatis personae largely in check, though recognizable when external triggers call them out – such as when they spontaneously act the fool, or adopt the teacher/preacher role, for example. Those whose inner world is inhabited with far more intense aspects of their personalities are likely to be ruled by them, such as Max illustrates. They serve an unconscious need to improve, sustain or protect a life situation. These are far more serious, driving the main persona in ways which at best can be unhealthy, at worst destructive.

Subpersonalities are forged in childhood, with the rest of the internal cast inhabiting the mysterious realms in the unconscious. To the outsider, phrases like Mummy's Boy or Daddy's Girl sound innocuous enough, conjuring up images of a doting mother, or of a proud father rejoicing in his pretty daughter. Actually, these pairings are seldom as they seem. A great deal of emotional blackmail, abuse and devouring are just as likely to be psychological backdrops to these family duos. Their fallout often lies behind a client's presenting problem, though they themselves will be unaware of the reason.

Therapists need to be alert to the fact that sitting in front of them one day might be a Petit Dauphin or Little Princeling; perhaps a Princess equally unable to grow up; a Benevolent Despot, convinced he must control his children for their own good; a Hero, come to save the day; a Judge, a Saboteur, a Scapegoat. The list is almost endless and practitioners will no doubt have their own fund of observations to identify these covert characters.

Perhaps the most poignant subpersonality is the Petit Dauphin, the Little Princeling, or as Jung called the eternal boy, *puer aeternus*. This subject, and its feminine counterpart, *puella aeterna*, is usefully discussed in the book by Jungian psychologist Marie-Louise von Franz (2000), *The Problem of the Puer Aeternus*, where she skilfully explains Jung's concept.

A Princeling takes the place of his physically or emotionally absent father and becomes the King to his mother's Queen as they go about their daily life. There is no question of his sexually moving into the role of consort. Usually the woman is not interested in sex, preferring the comfort of a devoted (and undemanding) son who will instead compliment, befriend her and act as confidant. When there is no psychologically functioning male on hand to act as a role model, the boy is in thrall to his mother, an unaware victim to her neediness. Often leading up to this, the boy will have had to work (probably unsuccessfully) through the Oedipal stage with her.

In the well-documented Oedipus phase, a little boy aged between three and five years unconsciously wants to possess his mother in an early libidinal development towards discovering his sexuality, and eliminate his father. So runs the psychoanalytical theory introduced by Freud at the beginning of the last century, borrowed from the Greek mythical story in which Oedipus unwittingly succeeds in marrying his mother and accidentally killing his father, with further terrible consequences. Freud suggests:

> ❝ His destiny moves us only because it might have been ours – because the oracle laid the same curse upon us before our birth as upon him. It is the fate of us all, perhaps, to direct our first sexual impulse towards our mother and our first hatred and our first murderous wish against our father.
>
> (1899: 296) ❞

Many therapists (and psychiatrists) today would disagree with this, yet we still hear echoes of the Oedipus story in session, no matter how obscure the presenting material might seem to blur this core issue. (The female version of the Oedipus complex applies to girls, of course, but we will return to this later.) How is the complex avoided all together? Put simply, in an emotionally healthy, functional home a little boy is rescued from his conflict of guilt and ambivalence by witnessing his father firmly (or metaphorically) close the marital bedroom door behind him, demonstrating then – and in his loving interaction with the mother – that he has sole claim.

A Princeling, on the other hand, usually has no psychologically functioning male to steer him to his own bedroom at the appropriate times; though he may be welcomed affectionately in the marital bed for morning cuddles and family fun. The unaware father either does not understand what is going on, in order to guide his son sensitively through the phase, or he may not even be there to see it.

Negative legacy

Moreover, in the dysfunctional home a father does not have to be physically absent to create a negative legacy for his son: many are the pitfalls awaiting a youngster if his parents' sexual life lacks vitality. When there is little or no intimacy, either in the relationship itself or behind the bedroom door, then unconsciously the boy will know this and the Oedipal phase remains a powerful energy still to be acknowledged. Later, it will go underground, as the boy grows up and forgets that early drive.

However, left unresolved and nurtured as in the case of the Little Princeling complex, his future relationships with women will almost inevitably suffer, often proving the underlying reason behind that particular partnership breakdown. Still bound to his mother, unable to find the penetrative thrust in his psychological make-up to cut loose from such dependency and go out into the world, he remains in a psychic prison, in many ways more boy than man. As Alix Pirani explains in *The Absent Father: Crisis and Creativity*:

66 The pain of this situation will be acute wherever wife and husband are not sufficiently 'together' because of his weakened potency or authority at home. There is no male succession in this structure: unless there is a work-area which is a shared male domain – i.e. a 'kingdom' – be it a family business or an accepted and mutually valued way of life for the men, then the negotiation for succession between father and son, needed as the son grows to manhood, cannot happen: it focuses instead on the regressive situation of the emotional relationship with the mother. So the father who could share

his own potency with his growing son, helping to empower him, instead uses his power to banish him, send him defence-less out into the world, or abandon him, defenceless to stand up to his overpowering mother.

(1988: 33–4) **99**

Sadly typical of the above scenario was William, a 38-year-old man recently made redundant from his job and needing some help to overcome depression. When we spoke about his mother he said:

66 She used to be strangely vague when I was about to leave school and think about what career to pursue. Whatever I wondered about doing, she'd clap her hands excitedly and say how good that would be, but I had absolutely no direction from her – she just enthused about the silliest ideas, and I was left floundering in doubt. My father never gave me any father–son talk, no linear thinking about what career I might achieve and enjoy, yet he was a university arts lecturer, quite able to discuss my options with the qualifications I had. There was always a sense of unease in our home, my mother often compensating for his silence in general and, frankly, becoming more with-drawn as life went on. Yes, I was stuck – I was her little prince in whom to confide and get masses of support. Of course I liked it, felt proud I could provide emotionally for her in the way my father could not. But it felt wrong somehow that I had to do this.

(personal communication) **99**

When William met Jane and they set up home together, their relationship began to falter as he found himself having to provide for both women. Jane resented the long telephone calls he was required to make with his mother, the over-frequent duty visits that were arranged behind her back. William's redun-dancy shock proved a turning point. The more Jane worried about lack of income, the more he retreated into his teenage daydreaming pattern. It was as if he was floating silly ideas for a fresh start in the same way he had with his mother, all those years ago. He was unconsciously pushing her to enthuse with current plans, however impractical, because therein lay the comfort of the familiar. He fully expected Jane to respond as his mother had done, celebrating the zany ideas, for despite the lack of incisiveness on her part she had always boosted his morale in the manner of reciprocal stroke giving. This time, William was not going to find an encouraging voice. Jane grew increasingly angry at his boyish, unrealistic ambitions. The partnership was in crisis. 'Grow up! Get real, William! I'm sick of your playing around with daft ideas – we need you to get a job, not live a dream,' said a desperate Jane, ready to leave him.

In therapy, William traced his life as stand-in for the absent King. He saw how the Queen, his mother, had abused their relationship by holding him to her for comfort and not releasing him to move on and find his own kingdom with a queen to love and cherish as his equal. There was a stagnancy about the entire family dynamic. Unless he could sever his attachment to the mother–son bond and create in time a new relationship with her, he would not be free to attend to the peer relationship with his wife. If his father had not reneged on his duty – to his wife, to his son – this static state of affairs might never have existed. As it was, William and Jane were locked into a new cell, in which the chances were odds on that any son of theirs would grow up to repeat much of the same pattern. Since no one had shown the way, how was William to know his own paternal responsibilities?

Not in good order

Most fathers adore their little girls, and most little girls rejoice in being adored by their father. Slave to their beguiling ways, an indulgent pushover for life, the majority of dads play out their protective role to everyone's satisfaction, where the male–female marital balance at home is in good order. But there is a category in the father–daughter relationship which is not in such good order, one which leaves a difficult legacy for the child involved. Often that daughter is highly intelligent, a bright girl who seems destined to walk a hazardous path with her equally bright father, particularly in later childhood and adolescence. She is Daddy's Princess.

Perhaps the reason for this lies in the fact that often a daughter finds her out-in-the-world identity first through Dad: this due to the double whammy sequence of development from the movement in the Oedipal stage (her first exploration of her sexuality) to the blossoming of her strong intellectual potential in which father – if also possessing a keen intellect – will revel. It is literally heady stuff, that heady energy locked at the mental level in an exciting secret bond. This constellation is beyond coincidence. I have seen it many times in the consulting room and believe the request for therapy is more often than not linked with that coincidence. Let us look at Laura's story:

CASE STUDY
Daddy's Princess

Laura came from a large family. She lacked maternal nurturing in that her mother was emotionally inaccessible, concerned with her own considerable career challenges. Her father, on the other hand, running a consultancy business from home, was available and always welcoming to his talented young daughter to talk over the day's events at school. As the years went on, they shared a common interest beyond academic talk – archaeology. Whenever the opportunity arose, they packed their bags and went abroad together to spend weeks away on various digs.

Laura by now had taken the place of her mother in all important aspects of a peer relationship, with the exception of the sexual component in a marriage. Neither of her parents was interested in sex, the erotic element long absent. Here, therefore, was a stagnancy in the marital situation (referred to in the Little Princeling dynamic) which induced a covert sexual energy. In turn this would lead to psychological dysfunction between father and daughter. Laura would become a long-term, inappropriate Daddy's Princess, his most cherished and desired female companion.

As Jungian analyst Marion Woodman explains in *The Ravaged Bridegroom*:

66 'Daddy's little princess' is the chosen child of her father. Blessed by his love, she may also be cursed by his love. Her special place in his dynasty sets her on a throne too remote for most princes to reach. Her throne is carved in ice, far from the nourishing warmth of Mother Earth. A father's daughter whose lifeline is to her dad may try to dismiss what is not there for her in her mother. Dad has been her cherishing mother and father. Why bother with what never was? If she decides to go into analysis, she will almost surely seek a male analyst because she respects men more than women and her energy is more vibrant with men. . . . A mother who cannot welcome her baby girl into the world leaves her daughter groundless. Similarly, the mother's mother and grandmother were probably without the deep roots that connect a woman's body to earth. Whatever the cause, her own instinctual life is unavailable to her and, disempowered as a woman, she runs her household as she runs herself – with shoulds, oughts and and have tos [sic] that add up to power. Life is not fed from waters of love but from will power that demands perfection, *frozen* perfection. Meanwhile, dad may in fact not be king but consort, so that father and daughter are unconsciously bonded against a tyrant queen – the mother as matriarch.

(1990: 73–4) 99

This observation neatly sums up Laura's background. Her mother was indeed undernourished emotionally, coming from a long line of achievers where the feminine qualities needed for balance were seriously lacking. It is likely her father discovered himself isolated – until his little daughter brought warmth and fun into his life.

Sexual energy may have gone underground, but it was still there, manifesting in giggly games when Daddy chased his young daughter round the room playing bears, hugging her too long, perhaps too closely when he caught her. In the Oedipal stage (when she was five or six) she basked in the adoring attention. It was, after all, her birthright to be encouraged towards discovering her sexuality. She relished being Daddy's Princess.

Then, as she grew towards puberty, the psychic seduction became less obvious (it had to be) and the intense emotional bond between them began to feel a dangerous trap for Laura. Their magical world together seemed now inexplicably shameful, though the 12-year-old girl was less likely to understand why. Her father, on the other hand, was aware – and alarmed – enough that he started to make fun of his daughter's changing body shape, to betray her trust in him by jeering at her tentative attempts to find a boyfriend.

Broken trust

So Laura not only had an absent and cold mother but now a taunting father, both parents seemingly only pleased with her when she produced glowing school reports. They approved of her taking his advice or direction because it was safe (for him) and a means to the desired academic end (for her). But Laura's sense of broken trust was profound. Where was the admiring Daddy, his loving acknowledgement of shared memories, the magical closeness she had once valued so much? Much later, as a bitter young woman she turned to a series of affairs with men who offered – at first sight – aspects of her father, in the way they adored her or admired her intellect. Inevitably, no one could match up to her unconscious needs for a return to blissful childhood.

As her second marriage began to falter, Laura realized she needed to explore the repeating pattern in her life, and she came into therapy. Dependent on alcohol for regular escapes into a safe hidden world, she was also bulimic. She looked thin and haggard, caught in a circular trap of bingeing, vomiting and drinking. 'I don't feel well,' she said one day. 'I know I look rubbish, but that's what it's all about, isn't it? I am feeding my belief I *am* rubbish: take biscuits and chocolate away, and I would have nothing left – I'd be an empty shell of uselessness.'

Laura spoke with awareness. Since her father had started showing his disapproval of her as she approached puberty, her self-confidence had faltered at a time in her development when she most needed his loving affirmation.

What she needed to hear – but did not get – were remarks to boost her sense of worth in this new arena of teenage discovery. This was the time in her life when she could have closed the book on her childhood secret bond, much as she might have put away her outgrown beloved toys. Not for her the warm acceptance, joyful celebration that his daughter had nearly grown up. Instead, and in their absence, Laura introjected the disapproving father (by unconsciously swallowing her father's disgust at himself and carrying his negative feelings into her own psyche) and began to see the world through his eyes.

She believed she had let her parents down, that she had failed to live up to their expectations in their clever daughter. No matter that her academic work reflected her high intelligence, she saw her school reports as markers of her inadequacies if there were not straight As in all subjects. She won a place at Oxford University and yet was baffled how she had done so. 'It must have been a fluke,' she said. The more she achieved, the more her father picked on what she had not achieved. 'Yes, that's all very well, but why didn't you publish a really important paper for your doctorate?' And so on.

Laura attracted plenty of male attention and found temporary respite from her unhappiness by enjoying the excitement of each fresh conquest. Up to a point, they reminded her of the thrill of travelling to a new dig with her father, the fun of shared interest. But her emptiness emotionally, somatized by her bulimia, always ended the relationship, disappointment evident on both sides. Laura was recreating the same scenario with her lovers as she experienced with her father in her teens. Paradoxically, she had to prove again and again that she was worthless, yet at the same time demanding of her boyfriends and marriage partners that they should be Daddy-like and treat her as a Princess. Jungians would call her a *puella aeterna*, the eternal girl (see Marie-Louise von Franz 2000). Until she could face her grief in therapy, reach the place of fear and powerlessness from which she had tried to escape since infancy, Laura could not gain psychological maturity.

To digress here for a moment, psychoanalyst Erik Erikson's theory of eight stages of psychosocial development come to mind. He suggests that the first stage – between birth and one year – is the most fundamental stage in life, where the child learns either trust or mistrust. Since the child is totally dependent, the development of trust will be based on the dependability of their caregivers' warmth, a reliable source of food and affection. Conversely, emotionally unavailable, inconsistent caring will create fear and insecurity in the baby, who will learn to see the world as unsafe, unpredictable, even dangerous. As Erikson movingly says in *Childhood and Society*:

> " Every adult, whether he is a follower or a leader, a member of
> a mass or of an elite, was once a child. He was once small. A
> sense of smallness forms a substratum in his mind, ineradi-
> cably. His triumphs will be measured against this smallness,

his defeats will substantiate it. The questions as to who is bigger and who can do or not do this or that, and to whom – these questions fill the adult's inner life far beyond the necessities and the desirabilities which he understands and for which he plans.

(1950: 404) **99**

So Laura, without that safe start in life, inevitably transferred her childhood dependence a few years later on to her father, who did offer warmth. However, she was to encounter yet more betrayal when she reached puberty. Decades later, she finally realized she needed help. Our work led to retracing the path back to the earliest days of her powerlessness, to infancy, to inhabit again the place in the inner world she most wished to resist. This meant hours of silent grief, of listening to the messages in her dreams as she experienced painful echoes of the anguish of her original abandonment, the sense of separateness, the terror. Then came the mourning over her father's betrayal. But as her therapy concluded she was ready to understand and forgive, recognizing that he too had lost a beloved companion in his beautiful little girl. Sadly, Laura's story is not unique – there are countless Daddy's Princesses out there, victims of emotional lacks and inherited ignorance.

Kindly tyrant

We have already seen that subpersonalities serve an unconscious need to improve or protect a life situation. When there is a strong neurotic urge to secure a sense of well-being by adopting a certain stance, or a presenting persona, then we see partners and families affected. Fear, low self-worth, under-confidence, insecurity can all lead to a need to control: the rationale being, of course, that if we take charge we stand less chance of further humiliation or loss. Many people hide their underlying reason for needing control over others by justifying their actions in the guise of 'knowing best', 'doing it for their own good', and so on. In reality, the Benevolent Despot is a tyrant, a control freak. Whether wife, husband, mother or father, in relationship with members of their family they exert a powerfully damaging influence, yet it is so subtle that influence appears kindness driven, a loving concern for everyone else but themselves.

A married man called Marcus illustrated this when he arrived to try to resolve his depression following redundancy from work. The more he talked about his sense of powerlessness, how ashamed he felt that he had let his parents down (no mention here of his wife and children), the more a picture developed about an over-controlled childhood. He was the son of a Benevolent Despot, where every move was judged but seldom applauded since he was a little boy. There was always a sting waiting to prick any minor or major achievement Marcus might have rushed home from school to announce, such as: 'Pity you couldn't have scored another goal at school today, they might have chosen you for the team.' So inured in believing his father's inflated self-evaluation of omniscience, Marcus had grown up to believe in that omniscience. He depended upon Dad's opinion in almost everything he did.

When he was made redundant, instead of coping as most people do, he collapsed. His concern was that he feared not so much about finding a new job but that he was disappointing his parents, now obviously much less a source of pride for them. Deeply depressed, he reviewed his life as a failure; this business setback surely proved it. Though a man in his early forties, he was still in the habit of asking his father for advice in writing job-search letters, uncertain of his own ability. Since the entire family acknowledged how clever Dad was with words, why make a mess of his own attempts when Dad could write so much better?

'What do you feel about that, really?' I asked.

'I know it might look as if Dad was treating me still as a child, but he *is* always right.'

'If anyone asked your father why he treats his son as if he were still a boy, what do you think his answer would be?'

'Almost certainly he would say it is his love for me that makes him take charge, of showing me how to get the best out of life . . . that love requires strict measures sometimes and that directing me will give me the benefit of his wisdom to enjoy it more. He did, after all, attend the University of Life, as he would say. He only wants the best for me,' and here his voice trailed off as the truth suddenly hit him. This was all about his father's need to feel good, his father's need for indirect glory, his father's need to feel indispensable.

Marcus risked a great deal later, when he decided this time not to ask for help writing job applications, thereby offending his mystified father. But at long last Marcus was moving away from the Benevolent Despot's control and began to take charge of his own life. His long-suffering wife welcomed the development as if he had been offered a huge pay rise. Now they could lead a normal life together, she declared, even if the going would be hard until a real new pay rise materialized.

Fundamental component

It would be inappropriate to claim here that subpersonalities such as those above are peculiar to specific types, or groups of people. They are not. We all have – to a greater or lesser degree – bits of them in our own psychic make-up, their strength of presence often depending on genes, environment, family belief systems and (most importantly) our early response to negative experience. Fear, therefore, is a fundamental component in the way that we unconsciously forge our various presenting personalities.

We may not have much of a presence, say, of the Benevolent Despot, but are we completely devoid of an inner Judge? Can we honestly say that there are not times when we assess another's behaviour; veer away from further contact with someone because they do not seem quite up to the mark in some way; secretly criticize what our friends or family do or do not do? Only when judging others becomes a way of life (such as adopted as essential practice by the parents of Marcus) could this and other subpersonalities be deemed neurotic. As we saw earlier, there is nothing too disruptive about the sudden appearance of a teacher, a comedian, a preacher. In their place, they can be helpful, instructive, or entertaining – and they soon go away again. Seldom entertaining and almost always frustrating to others, however, is the Saboteur. This subpersonality (if resident) tends to be a fixture in someone's psyche. Appearing in subtle unconscious manoeuvres, always concerned with warding off potentially frightening situations ahead, the Saboteur has great power precisely because his or her means of achieving avoidance is hard to pinpoint.

It all seems so plausible: a husband, frightened his wife will stay permanently away on a solitary trip suddenly discovers a serious medical condition requiring her to drive him immediately to hospital and stay with him; a lover, guilty about an illicit meeting, wakes up that morning to discover his lumbar region requires an urgent visit to the osteopath (is he 'backing out' for fear of reprisal?); a gifted student unaccountably fails her examinations, so ensuring she need not leave home.

It often seems the physical body is the vehicle through which the Saboteur can secure a successful outcome (for its own needs). What is fascinating is how that comes about. Was the genuine medical condition just a coincidence, yet manifesting crucially on the day a restless wife planned her long-distance trip? Did the crippling backache, normal eight hours earlier yet excruciating next morning, provide an acceptable 'torpedo' to cancel the secret rendezvous, while not completely closing the door on a future meeting? We are reminded here of Hillman's remarks in *The Soul's Code* about our daimon's ability to protect, invent or even make the body ill (1996: 39).

Once again too we are witness to the extraordinary power of our unconscious minds. The link between body and mind is now acknowledged, both in orthodox medicine and in the holistic world. But if we consider the examples here, the precise timing involved and the obedient somatic response which would most serve the Saboteur – well, here it deserves top billing for cunning. Yes, it functions like the ally (or daimon) does, organizing scenarios for a good outcome; the difference being, however, that a healthy result for the subject's overall well-being is not the Saboteur's goal. Its clever avoidance strategies are merely to keep the subject out of trouble. The long-term view does not seem important, much as it might not to a child or adolescent. Perhaps we could reason that the job of healing is unintentionally left to the ally in the unconscious, waiting for the right time, right place to bring about change.

Two more examples: a female client announced she was considering taking part-time employment where, as ever, she feared the possibility of not being good enough. It was a lucrative job and she needed work. She said, 'Of course, my recurrent migraines make it impractical to commit to full-time. I wouldn't want to seem unreliable by needing to take a day off sick most weeks.' What she was saying, unaware, was that her Saboteur had 'arranged' migraine attacks whenever she did not feel on top of the job requirement and that falling ill in the past was her only way of bypassing humiliating confrontations with her line manager. Not realizing the significance of that strategy over many years, now she simply wanted to plan a schedule that would ensure recovery time without embarrassment.

She believed she was martyr to painful headaches due to chemical imbalance or an inherited weakness. When asked if she could remember the onset of the first ever migraine she answered, 'Day One of my job after qualifying as a designer. And then, any evening before a work presentation day.' Still she could see no pattern emerging, yet the message was evident: she was unconsciously worried she would be found wanting and she feared a showdown.

These migraines, of course, had implication too in the quality of the relationship with her husband. He was sympathetic at first, then frustrated at the regularity of the headaches. By the time the underlying problem had surfaced and been discussed in session, my client realized how much her hidden drive to keep out of trouble was seriously jeopardizing the relationship, as well as compromising employment prospects. So began useful work on all of it. The daimon/ally had trumped the Saboteur, nudging my client towards resolution.

Why this is not always the case – that the daimon had superimposed its will over a powerful subpersonality – is unanswerable. We cannot know, we cannot guess. Once again, we bow to the imponderable and wait for enlightenment, new research or new insight.

Driven to drink

The second example is brief but telling. A recovering alcoholic, who knew his hated elderly mother would need his care once she was out of hospital following a stroke, dreaded the prospect and began drinking again to dull the feelings. Two years earlier, the man had been caught drink-driving, and was heavily fined along with penalty points. Warned any further offence would be viewed much more seriously, he nonetheless took his car out the morning after a bout of heavy drinking. He was caught by the police.

'This will mean prison for me,' he announced, convinced this would be his fate. During our session, the client admitted that a spell in prison, however unpleasant, would be preferable to looking after his mother; that would now be someone else's task, other arrangements would have to be made. His

Saboteur had gone to extraordinary lengths to ensure he was locked up, away from maternal demands. Only as we looked more closely at the recklessness involved in taking a car on the road when he knew he was still drunk did understanding dawn. 'Yes,' he said, shaking his head in amazement, 'that is exactly what I did to avoid a worse sentence indoors with my mother.'

There is one last subpersonality we should introduce here in the line-up of the most common dramatis personae dwelling in our unconscious world. That subpersonality is called the Scapegoat. Often the middle born, but by no means always, a little child will learn quickly that his or her role in the family is to bear the blame, responsibility, worry or whatever. We could describe them as the Sin Eaters, echoing the Aztec goddess's gift of devouring people's inner blackness to cleanse them.

It is a role accepted easily by certain personality types – usually the affable, gentle, compliant member who, in the normal family, will be boisterously taken advantage of by more assertive siblings. But here we are concerned with a darker side to this scenario, where fear or even borderline pathology drives blaming and culpability towards the original concept of sin eating. The Scapegoat tends to bear the burden – or is the butt of – others' neuroses.

Then there is the 'naughty child' example of Scapegoat, whose only intuitive means of drawing attention to the dysfunctional dynamic in the family is to act out the underlying disturbance, such as in losing their temper, passionately and frequently. This behaviour is not to be confused with everyday childhood outbursts, where the child is on a learning curve, trying and testing their boundaries. In older children, though, inexplicable rages might point to their overall unease in the home environment. No one else can, or is likely to be able to, identify and own the family dysfunctionalism: it has fallen to this one member unconsciously to express it for them.

I have known of distressing cases where a youngster tries their best to make Mum and Dad happier together, not just to win their love and approval but to make life at home more tolerable for everyone. One small boy, realizing how his parents quarrelled about most things, including housework, found a way (as he imagined) to quell the bickering: he polished all the kitchen, bathroom and basin taps until they gleamed. Nobody noticed. So he went on doing it, still hoping for family peace. Of course, when he grew up he continued his role as Scapegoat, always taking the blame either directly or indirectly for tense atmospheres in the home, at the office, or with friends. He reasoned that the fact of his parents' disharmony ending in divorce must have been his fault: he should have tried harder. For him, there never would be an end to his self-imposed belief. He carried the world's badness on his shoulders, Sin Eater for all. Disabling illness eventually put a stop to that. It was as if he had wearied of the task to make things better for people, despair turning in on itself, with his body somatizing his anger and exhaustion after never getting it right for others.

Summary

Clues to discovering the core issues in a client's presenting problem will often lie in identifying their operating subpersonalities. Those whose internal world is inhabited with intense aspects of their predominant subpersonalities are likely to be ruled by them. They serve as an unconscious need to improve or protect a life situation; and these are far more serious than the everyday joker, teacher or preacher, for example, who appear temporarily on cue to certain external triggers.

Where a subpersonality has become embedded in the psyche for the purpose of defending against further hurt (imagined or real), it is much more substantial; it drives the main personality in ways which are at best unhealthy, at worst destructive. It can affect relationships bewilderingly – a partner, or offspring, cannot be expected to understand the powerful influence of these second-in-line hidden operators at work – and will sometimes reach a state of despair.

Only when therapy or counselling is recognized as a solution to unravel the knots will a couple or individual have the chance to learn to change that powerful influence, whether in themselves or in having been on the receiving end of parents' influences years before. First, they will need help to spot the ruling subpersonality, precisely because these characteristics grow slowly, subtly over the years according to the environment in which the child was brought up.

Asking clients to talk about their childhood (open questions being the most useful approach, gently pursuing the quality of feelings emerging as they recount their stories) can yield important clues to pinpoint likely subpersonalities directing their life. Since fear is almost always behind this, the therapeutic work must focus on discovering the core issues and then new ways of breaking away from their grip.

Clients may often be resistant to accepting the truth of their upbringing, that same upbringing which caused such catastrophic impact and about which they may well be in denial. Care must be taken, therefore, to ensure they do not feel disloyal to parents in revealing their past, thus blocking the road to healing. It often helps the process forward to assure them in session that nobody is to blame. We are all – to a greater or lesser extent – casualties of our environment. Most parents really did do their best, victims themselves no doubt to earlier defensive means unconsciously devised by previous generations.

In the next two chapters we will look at the difficulties (and triumphs) experienced by certain categories of adult partnerships, where childhood, genes and environmental factors had major impact on the quality of their future relationships.

4 Couples with 'normal neurotic' disorders

A glance at the lexicon of psychiatric disorders – from obsessional compulsive behaviour to paranoia – could convince us that almost everyone we know is clinically ill, much as medical students identify for themselves worrying symptoms of serious disease when they study their textbooks. But the following is about 'normal neurotic', or 'the worried well', who make up most adults in our day-to-day world; folk who by no means qualify as outpatients in a mental hospital, disabled by their illness. We are talking about ordinary people we work with, who live next door (or with us) and, indeed, about ourselves.

As we have already seen, there are bits of personality types, subpersonalities and character structures in everyone. Much will depend on the mix of genetic predisposition, nurture, or the lack of it, and a host of other factors. Founder of bioenergetics therapy Alexander Lowen has this to say about the reasons behind our defensive development:

> The primary orientation of life is toward pleasure and away from pain. This is a biological orientation, because on a body level, pleasure promotes the life and being of the organism. Pain, as we all know, is experienced as a threat to the organism's integrity. We open up and reach out spontaneously to pleasure, and we contract and withdraw from a situation that is painful. When, however, a situation contains a promise of pleasure, coupled with a threat of pain, we experience anxiety. . . . Pavlov's work on conditioned reflexes in dogs clearly demonstrated how anxiety could be produced by combining in one situation a painful stimulus with a pleasurable one. . . . The dog was in a bind, wanting to move toward the food but afraid to do so, and so was thrown into a state of severe anxiety.
>
> This pattern of being placed in a bind by mixed signals is the cause of the anxiety underlying all neurotic and

psychotic personality disorders. The situations that lead to the bind occur in childhood between parents and children. Babies and children look to parents as a source of pleasure and reach out to them with love. This is the normal biological pattern, since parents are the source of food, contact and sensory stimulation that infants and children need. Until it meets with frustration and suffers deprivation, an infant is all core – that is, heart.

(1975: 135–6) **99**

Lowen, concerned as he is with body work, focuses upon the ultimate splitting that results from a lifelong struggle to defend against further pain while still functioning from mind and heart. He would argue that the body reflects the disassociation – in different ways according to the personality of the individual, determined, as he says, by his vitality – that is, by the strength of his impulses and by the defences he has erected to control these impulses. 'No two individuals are alike in either their inherent vitality or in their patterns of defence arising from their life experience. Nevertheless, it is necessary to speak in terms of types for the sake of clarity in communication and understanding,' he adds (1975: 151).

Emotionally unavailable

Backing up the point, Pulitzer prizewinner Erik Erikson, one of the last century's leading figures in the field of psychoanalysis and human development, writes in *Childhood and Society* that caregivers in a baby's first year who are inconsistent, emotionally unavailable or who reject them in some way create a basic mistrust in the child. Conversely, mothers who provide a sense of trust by combining sensitive care of the baby's individual needs give the child a firm sense of identity which will later combine a sense of being 'all right', of being oneself, and of becoming what other people trust they will become. He goes on:

66 The absence of basic trust results in a lifelong underlying weakness, apparent in adult personalities in whom withdrawal into schizoid and depressive states is habitual. The reestablishment of a state of trust has been found to be the basic requirement for therapy in these cases . . . [Defence] mechanisms are, more or less normally, reinstated in acute crises of love, trust, and faith in adulthood and can characterize irrational attitudes towards adversaries and enemies in masses of 'mature' individuals.

(1950: 248–9) **99**

We are discussing, however, the people who live on our street, with whom we work, or with whom we live. We know dozens in our own circles, family, friends, associates, for **schizoid** people are legion. They are those men and women whose early emotional traumas caused a splitting off, a non-presence similar to 'sitting on the fence' when they encounter difficulties. Unlike psychologist Arthur S. Reber's clinical definition of schizoid personality disorder, which he says is characterized by 'a lack of interest in social relationships, a tendency towards a solitary lifestyle, secretiveness, and emotional coldness' (1995: 690), a normal neurotic schizoid has, seemingly, none of these tendencies.

On the contrary, they often appear at their happiest in a warm circle of friends, sharing confidences, eager to be included. Yet underlying this there is a detectable hidden layer of self which is ready to flee, to peel away from contact. Their detachment can be devastating to a partner who will find the steely separateness unbearable, particularly when their own emotional furnace is on fire with the urgency to try to resolve a dispute. So adept at splitting off are schizoid folk that they feel virtually nothing – and that remains true for those moments.

Early life trauma, usually associated with poor quality nurturing, taught the otherwise powerless child to avoid any further stress by taking their minds somewhere else. No matter how much in adult life their partner might plead for them to engage with them, respond to points raised and 'come back' once more, they seem unable to do so. Sounds familiar? Watch the expression change on the schizoid's face when attack, or some other kind of emotional danger (real or imagined) looms. Their eyes lose contact, feeling, they look through rather than at you. The entire energetic system has gone away. Nathan Field explains it succinctly (and a touch more sympathetically than Erikson does):

> 66 Each of us, in infancy, resorts to these defensive mechanisms in order to mitigate the intense pain that inevitably comes with being an infant. According to Fairbairn (1952: 3–27) we are all, at the deepest level, schizoid. Put more provocatively: none of us is normal. . . . However empathic our parenting, since it cannot be perfect, none of us can quite escape becoming schizoid: that is, we defensively split off into the unconscious a part of our personality and lose our primary wholeness.
>
> (1996: 128–9) 99

Of course, we could draw a parallel here with full-blown schizophrenia, where profound splitting creates at first sight a not dissimilar set of presenting symptoms. But this is not the case when we consider this particular character type here. Degrees of trauma are relative, as we already know from Walker's observations about multiple personality disorder. Walker explains that the condition arises as an 'extreme response to equally extreme multiple abuse' (1992: 113). In the schizoid type we usually learn of much less extreme abuse (in the widest sense), where a sensitive child cannot cope with the confusing, unreliable quality of their environment.

The traumas of infancy apart, this might stem from loneliness, a sense of being unloved or conditionally loved, perhaps of being the least favoured member of the family, a failure at coping with bullying at school (by that age the pattern will already have been set but compounded by this extra stress), even being exceptionally gifted, dyslexic, dyspraxic. The schizoid child finds life's difficulties unbearable; they learned in infancy to switch off, to pretend they were not there, and the habit has stuck. In therapy, they might refer to 'sitting on the fence looking on at life', of 'retreating up a mountain', of 'singing songs in their head' whenever their emotional well-being seems in danger.

Yet in adult life the schizoid man or woman will be – to the outside world – highly functional and capable of dealing with any amount of adult decision making. The problem manifests when their personal relationship (usually with their partner, unconsciously representing the original carer) hits trouble, as we have already seen from Erikson. Then they quit the scene, physically present, emotionally departed. Fairbairn describes it thus: 'The individual begins to tell us that he feels as if there was nothing to him, or as if he had lost his identity, or as if he were dead, or as if he had ceased to exist' (1952: 3–27).

Complementary opposites

Now let us consider a child offering a very different make-up, not necessarily less sensitive but perhaps more genetically programmed to stay with the pain rather than flee. This child will be a candidate for future anxiety states, rather than withdrawal or depression. Her or his legacy of a less than perfect infancy will show itself in worry, hysteria, sometimes uncontrollable passionate outbursts, by the time they have grown up. Fully present, more grounded than psychologically sitting on the fence, and not one bit disassociated from what is going on, the **histrionic** type is in fact the complementary opposite to the schizoid structure. When their relationship works, it can prove a creative and mutually healing partnership. When their relationship fails, it brings great suffering.

The histrionic (or previously called hysteric) was once seen by Freud as a penis-envying, sexually dysfunctional woman. This outdated view was adapted and developed by Wilhelm Reich in the 1940s and then much more clearly presented by psychoanalyst Alexander Lowen. In his book *The Language of the Body*, Lowen says:

> ❝ The hysterical attack is the psychic counterpart of the attempt to repress a strong anxiety state. Freud recognized the corollary of this proposition when he said (1894a, page 105) that, 'aspects come to light which suggest that anxiety neurosis is actually the somatic counterpart of hysteria'. The hysterical attack is an explosive phenomenon. The sudden development of an excess of energy can overwhelm the ego in a so-called hysterical outburst, or it can be funneled into one part of the body and isolated, their [sic] producing an hysterical symptomatology.
>
> (1958: 255) ❞

Hence the incidence of hysterical paralysis, where a client may report suddenly losing the use of her arms, hands or legs during an emotional tirade. But psychoanalysis moved on again and now describes such a client as histrionic which, taken to pathological level, is characterized by an excessive emotionality and need for approval.

Where the Greek word for womb (*hystera*) had its root in Freud's definition (the reason obvious), over the past century we have embraced latterly the Latin *histrionicus* for the root – that of being an actor, or of histrionically putting on a showy act. I am inclined to stay with the former for the type under discussion. In the 'normal neurotic' band, such clients fit more neatly into Lowen's description, as the following case study (Anthony and Clare) may illustrate.

Where the schizoid partner will continue to feel next to nothing as the relationship ends (he or she having stayed locked in their split-off mental retreat), the damage to the emotionally overflowing histrionic, or hysteric, mate will be great. This is their tragedy: where one cannot reach the other, little can be done to retrieve a faltering situation. However, we might throw some light here on how all need not be lost when this state of impasse occurs.

CASE STUDY
Couple in crisis

Anthony and Clare presented in therapy as a couple in crisis. Money worries, a disastrous business transaction hovering like a black cloud over the future had called out their worst characteristics respectively. The more Clare wept tears of frustration and anger, the more Anthony emotionally absented himself. His eyes gave the impression of seeing from a million miles away; his body was still, hands folded, almost as if he had packed himself into a perspex box, oblivious to her tears. Clare cried out, 'You see? This is what I get all the time at home – he just refuses to engage with me. But I'm telling him really important things, facts he needs to hear, if we're to get out of our money difficulties. I feel so alone, so unheard.'

Asked to comment, Anthony replied, 'She's just being hysterical. There's no real need to get so upset about our financial difficulties – something will turn up. Clare is being completely over the top about this: she won't trust me, keeps nagging, nagging, nagging. No wonder I close down.' Here was a major block. Her heartfelt statement about feeling alone and unheard was never going to be understood by a man whose own survival belief lay in the need to take care of himself, by himself, as far away as possible.

Trust was of course a huge issue for Anthony. In the early stages of therapy he often said he could not trust Clare (citing one wintry occasion when, at the peak of marital frustration, she had demanded he leave their house in the early hours, with nowhere for him to go in a car which had a near-empty tank). Betrayal was equally a major issue for Clare. She expected Anthony to look after her, to rescue her from their crises just as her father had in her teens, referring to his daughter as his Little Princess. Anthony called her a screaming banshee. Clare saw him as an insensitive monster. In one key therapy session I offered the following:

> 66 It seems to me we can either agree he's a monster, Clare, and that you are a banshee, or we consider the fact that it's unlikely you'd both be together after so long if these charges were actually true. What I think we are hearing through these harsh words is really your ancient fear and anger – on both sides. Clare is distressed and forceful about her case and Anthony is feeling cut off, sad he can't ever get it right. Clare's frantic neediness polarizes Anthony into a far corner, in that the more outraged she becomes at what she considers his failures to deliver, the more Anthony retreats, not out of cowardice but a real sense of impotence: classic flawed early relationship. Blaming, right-and-wrong stuff isn't getting us anywhere. We need to look at what's really behind this impasse between you both. It feels as if two hurt children are offloading, perhaps for the first time expressing fully wounds that once as little people neither could possibly have articulated. Your rage belongs to decades ago, but present events have restimulated or reinstated it. 99

Crucially, as we explored their respective early lives, we learned that Anthony's sensitivity was too great to bear the emotional unpredictability of his upbringing: hence a desensitivity to any future resonating encounters. The first casualty came almost inevitably with his first marriage, as did Clare's. In her case, a single child with an alcoholic mother, she depended on support from her father in compensation. When he died, she went searching to replace him, only to be disappointed in her first marriage but finding something of her father in Anthony's charming, capable and talented ways when she met him as a divorcee in her forties. We could say that their unconscious allies magnetized them to each other – for there was reparation to be done.

Why did Anthony survive his childhood by splitting off and Clare remain down to earth and emotionally accessible, despite similar traumas? There cannot be a simple answer, since we know in considering the human psyche that we are dealing with the multifactorial, where genetic predisposition, siblings – or lack of them – support systems other than maternal, illness, and so on all need to be taken into account. Perhaps Clare's initial mothering was good enough in those vital early stages of bonding, only to deteriorate as her carer became unreliable. Having a consistently loving father, however, provided sufficient security to carry her through to adult autonomy. But the early scars were still in need of healing.

Anthony's history programmed him differently, though he too achieved adult autonomy. Perhaps his arrival as a baby was compromised in some way. His father certainly was emotionally and physically absent and when his mother died a few years later Anthony had to seek a measure of affection from a series of nannies. Later at school he threw himself into camaraderie with boys and sport. When he met Clare, however, he fell deeply in love. They lived together for many years, clearly enjoying each other's company, pooling their creative skills, complementary to each other as they opened and ran a string of retail shops. Yet here in the therapy room was a near breakdown of their long relationship, now that serious business crisis loomed.

It was clear that each was dealing with their current stress according to the predominant survival methods: Anthony as schizoid, Clare as histrionic/hysteric. Deep hurt lay behind their relationship clash yet neither recognized it. His armoury relied on splitting off from the painful moment, hers in staying angrily present, determined to reach him with a pyrotechnic display of fiery words. The more she raged, the more he disappeared.

Invited in session to talk about her lonely childhood, Clare described an alcoholic mother who had little time for her. Each morning before breakfast, Clare worried about the mood she might have to cope with – being shouted at or being ignored. Naturally, this set up a hunger for attention, for a carer who would be interested in her daily world, to give encouragement and support. She built her own world, playing shops and making pretty things for her father to admire when he came home after work. Small wonder Clare expected similar attention from Anthony and when she was unhappy, for him to hear her pain and loneliness; and small wonder her increasingly frantic demands were met with stony deafness.

(Another schizoid client I have worked with called Robert once likened his shut off feelings when under supposed 'attack' to being a tortoise, where instant reflex takes over before the mind can reason away the cause. He explained, 'It is to do with safety, when the tortoise withdraws his head and neck and hides under his carapace away from harm. I view it also like that instinct to shut our eyes when a stone or flying paper hits the windscreen as we're driving, and no matter how much we know that neither will actually hit our face, we flinch.')

In post-therapy feedback several years later, Clare said, 'I was getting so hysterical when Anthony failed to understand me, I wasn't using my intellect. Fear stopped me seeing what was really going on. Because my mother had been so self-absorbed, whenever Anthony shut down on me it was terrifying – it was just like I experienced life with her.' She added:

> Therapy taught me to stand back and look at the situation from the outside, which lessened the hysteria. I slowly began to see him as a very kind man, with a much softer side to him – not someone to fear. I learned too that it's okay to say 'no', and not to be a people pleaser to make me feel I wasn't such a bad person, all my ancient stuff from childhood. As I grew to trust Anthony, those self-esteem issues melted away: I'd always wanted a 'rock' for a partner and now our financial crises are largely over can see that together as a partnership and as a working team, we are as capable as any of getting through any amount of horrors life throws at us. We are much more balanced as a pair. I use my creativity better in our work, and he feels safer to discuss sensitive areas like finance. It's as if somebody had put something into a glass of water and suddenly the colour changed – that's how I now see my emotional life with Anthony. And it feels great!
>
> (personal communication)

Anthony said:

> Talking in front of our therapist without interruptions, as we'd all agreed, no rows permitted, I understood better what lay under my own grievances. We had in fact both come through awkward home lives, isolated from other kids because of our difficult mothers. There is a logic why someone reacts a certain way to triggers, therefore an explanation of our background and history has had a big impact on my realizing how we handle things. Dealing with areas of contention nowadays

have been softened, and we are much more adept at avoiding head-on clashes simply by understanding a lot of the reasons behind those clashes. There is a level of acceptance now [in me] that there are some differences in our lives which are not really going to change – practical, financial considerations, our children from other marriages and their different needs, and the fact that Clare will continue to get over-emotional. I still shut off because I believe her 'screaming' doesn't achieve anything, if other attempts at resolution haven't worked this time. Yes, I am resigned to those differences, but as Clare herself has said, we have discovered a relationship glue that holds us together now, as never before.

(personal communication) 99

This maturity in their joint view makes a useful illustration to support Jungian analyst James Hall's comment in his book *The Jungian Experience*:

66 In conventional marriage or couple therapy the focus is too often on the decision of whether to stay together or to separate, whereas the real *process* that is involved is the maturation of one or both of the partners. Since this is never exactly a balanced situation – both parters are never at precisely the same growth point – it requires careful understanding of the processes in *both* to do justice to the underlying potentialities in each of them. Jung discussed the problems of relationship in an important essay 'Marriage as a Psychological Relationship'. The greater the extent of unconsciousness in one or both of the partners, he suggested, the less is marriage a matter of free conscious choice (*Collected Works* 17 para. 327). For one thing, if a person is unconscious of the actual conflicts that disturb him or her, the 'cause' is *frequently projected on to the partner*.

(1986: 113, my italics) 99

This says it all. We shall see time and again just how often projection creates so much pain in personal relationships – and how vital it is for therapists and counsellors to appreciate and work with this aspect of the theory of projection. Our childhood draws us to our adult partners; and it will also destroy them unless the necessary excavation work is done. Unconscious fears, hurts, hopes and expectations invariably lie behind our choice of mate and the subsequent conflict or disappointment we meet. Statistics of marital breakdown would suggest the truth of this. But Clare and Anthony's story comes along to encourage a belief that talking therapy can reverse the trend.

Subtle sabotage

So far we have looked at the schizoid and the hysteric types in this discussion on working with couples presenting with normal neurotic disorders. There are, of course, many other character structures which could enter this arena – such as oral, masochistic, narcissistic – but I have chosen to write about the most commonly seen pairings, where one or other has a disorder which threatens the quality of relationship, one which will exacerbate the projection problems. There is one group in society where it is harder to identify precisely which 'normal neurotic' disorder they fall into or suffer from (or more accurately, their partner) and this is to be discovered in the **passive aggressive** type.

Basically afraid to confront (the timorous child who never found their angry voice), passive aggressive folk live much of their life being indirect. They will say 'Oh, I don't mind what we do/where we go/whatever time suits you.' Yet, after someone has made a decision by default, they will as like as not overhear the sulky comment, 'We won't get home until late if we do such and such' or 'Of course, he's not my favourite actor, but if that's who you want to see, we'll go to that film.' And so on.

It is frustrating to deal with as a family member, and equally so to pinpoint as a counsellor or therapist. Every suggestion that indirect behaviour might be getting in the way of sensible resolution tends to be met with innocent, even indignant reaction. A passive aggressive man or woman is unconsciously intent on getting what he or she wants without sticking their neck above the psychological parapet. Their need above all is to avoid confrontation, instead to be seen as blameless, peaceful, accommodating. Their childhood almost certainly provided no opportunity to express rage (often suppressed by controlling parents or bullying siblings) and this would have led to devising other means of making their point or hitting back. The habit followed them seamlessly into adulthood, when they would unconsciously choose powerful mates, replicating the familiar interaction. What at first seemed welcome consideration to a husband, proud of his easy-going wife, would sooner or later take on a subtle change.

'Rebecca is driving me mad with frustration!' burst out Rebecca's irate spouse in an early therapy session. 'She'll never be on time for an outing, if she doesn't really want to go. By the time she's ready, the party or whatever is nearly over and so she has actually controlled the evening and upset the host. She would totally deny that, pointing regretfully at urgent telephone calls she was obliged to answer, and then end the row with a sorrowful comment on my wish to make an issue of her lateness, when she was doing her best to cope with other problems. She loathes making decisions, or firm commitments and yet she will quietly complain about others' inability to do the same when it affects her own plans.'

Invited to offer her take on Luke's outburst, Rebecca said firmly, 'I don't believe in angry rows, it is morally indefensible. I didn't intend to get delayed by the 'phone calls, but they were important. Luke is being very unreasonable in saying I deliberately delayed getting ready. I try my best to be accommodating to everyone, and I can't bear these outbursts of his. It's really so unfair, just when I'm trying to do the best I can for everyone.'

This sugar sweet attitude did not ring true, though I would never have challenged her at this juncture – Rebecca would be the first to cancel the next booked session with a plausible excuse that put her, the martyr, in a righteous position which was unassailable. She would probably have used passive aggression at the therapist (away from me) by reminding her husband at home that the sessions were costly and they could surely work out their problems on their own without all this expense.

So I said nothing. The couple continued coming for some weeks. But once Rebecca (who had assumed she had won over the therapist to her point of view) began to hear the beginnings of confrontation instead, she did exactly what I had guessed she would do: she persuaded her husband the sessions were not working for them. Poor Luke.

What if the therapy had worked? It would have required Rebecca identifying and taking responsibility for her behaviour as a strategy to get her way without unpleasantness, accepting that as a child she had used indirect methods for fear of reprisal if she had vented her real feelings. It would also have meant Luke learning to challenge her immediately he suspected she was controlling from a passive place; to encourage her to enter a more communicative arena, quarrelling if necessary as they looked at reality together instead of his unwillingly having to swallow her plausible excuses for controlling, or sulky resentment whenever he did fight his corner.

Confrontation is a risky business, and asking someone in this behaviour category to alter habits of a lifetime is a daunting task. Remember, in childhood they were probably traumatized when innocently confronting their parents or siblings; their memory will steer them to avoid at all costs the danger of further trauma. But sympathy and encouragement from their spouse to take risks as never before could prove rewarding.

Escaping anxiety

Superstition, ritual, even religion is seen the world over as a legitimate means to feel better and avoid existential anxiety: of death, exclusion, punishment, failure, disempowerment, what you will. But for some, there is no formulaic method to ward off the terrors of the night (or day). Unconsciously, they decide they must work something out for themselves. Enter the **obsessive compulsive**, or the person who is driven to carry out bizarre rituals to ward off what they irrationally believe threatens them (obsessive compulsive disorder, OCD). They are aware their behaviour carries no logic. They fear, for example, contracting disease from doorknobs, so they wash their hands frequently, yet they cheerfully face a parachute jump or water skiing without regard to their safety.

What of the effect compulsive perfectionism has upon a relationship? It can be hard work, irritating and downright infuriating, as client Cheryl explained. Her husband Clive washes his hands dozens of times a day, even more frequently when he has been out of the home, imagining he has brought back a dangerous disease picked up from opening or shutting public doors. He goes round the house at night checking that the cooker has been turned off, that windows and doors are all locked safely – and then not only double checks, but performs that night watch at least six times daily.

66 He gets no pleasure from doing any of those things – that is, he gets no sense of security to have checked locks so many times. He goes to bed still worrying, and that leaves me obviously picking up some of his anxiety too. There's nothing relaxed and comfortable about living with Clive, even though I love him dearly. I find he constantly needs reassurance that I did witness him checking on safety; he can be quite like a young child, emotionally clinging on to me for safety.

Once I inherited some beautiful designer clothes from a dear friend who had died of cancer. Despite all the medical evidence to the contrary, Clive saw those clothes as potentially infective and he insisted I give them away to a charity shop. I was really upset about this, and we had lots of heartbreaking rows about it. Eventually, I came to be reconciled with the fact that I lived with someone with OCD and that I had either to accept his irrational fears, or leave him. He's far too lovely to do that.

(personal communication) 99

Four generations (at least) of women in one family suffered from the condition which – 50 years ago – would once have been seen as worthy rather than sad. Sally's grandmother ran a market garden business with her husband, kept an immaculate house and never set foot outside her domain, no doubt regarded by the neighbours as an ultra-devoted wife and mother. Her daughter (Sally's mother) in due course found it impossible to climb on to a bus in order to visit Sally when she was newly married, in desperate need of help as she herself struggled with obsessional fear. Now her own daughter has been diagnosed with the condition.

Is this a case of inherited genes, or did each female unconsciously learn to fear by watching their OCD mother's behaviour, or was it a case of predisposition exacerbated by nurture? No researcher yet has found the definitive answer. Meanwhile, Sally and her husband lead a constrained life, unable to invite friends to dinner (Sally is afraid the food might spoil) or, on a wider scale, to plan adventurous family holidays, limited to return year after year to the same safe, familiar place.

Sally sought help for her primary school daughter, realizing the problems lying ahead if the disorder gripped the youngster as badly as it had her. In family therapy, Sally was told that she held the answer to overcoming the condition. 'The only person to help you is yourself,' she was told by a cognitive behaviour therapy practitioner, 'with encouragement from a professional to guide you along the way. We can remind you, challenge you, about the avoidance strategies you use so as not to have to put yourself through the misery of doing things you fear. But you and your daughter need to take responsibility, not let the condition control you.'

Psychotherapist James Hillman holds the view that 'obsessions be given courtesy' (1996: 161). In *The Soul's Code* he suggests that a child needs to be respected when he or she is at play, in the middle of a mess or running wild through the bushes: the child puts into play the germinal code [of his destiny] that pushed it into these obsessive activities. Repression of this, where parents require their child to conform to their own fantasy of how they should behave, might 'return full flood into him . . . his language, his habits. . . . For it is not ultimately parental control or parental chaos that children run away from; they run from the void of living in a family without any fantasy beyond shopping, keeping up the car, and routines of niceness.'

We might accept this singular view as a valuable insight into one causative factor behind clients with obsessional compulsive disorder: that is, where some distortion or suppression (once imposed upon natural behaviour) created in the child a deep anxiety, manifested in later life in non-related repetitive devices, unconsciously to try to ensure only good happens. Their childhood behaviour (developing skills in play, fantasy in timeless concentration, though misunderstood or unappreciated by their primary carers) could have produced countless high achievers in the world of sport, the arts, science and politics, their achievements enhanced by these early patterns.

Fear everywhere

It is a fact of the human condition that fear – in all its guises – can and does determine the quality of the life that we lead. As we have already seen, it drives the schizoid, the histrionic, the passive aggressive and the obsessive compulsive types to function at the level in their personality best adapted to cope with their world and its conflicts. Thus far, we have looked at problems encountered in relationships where some form of dysfunctional behaviour has been unconsciously adopted to defend the owner from further pain. But there is a final category here where fear cannot as easily be utilized, because fear itself is the presenting problem. Living with someone who struggles with dread can be a heavy burden and put a huge strain on the relationship.

People who suffer from paranoia, phobias and panic attacks lead an unenviable life, their fearful imagination giving rise to countless nightmare scenarios. Though fear lies behind every manifestation, irrationality and suspiciousness probably describe best the 'normal neurotic' level of the disorder called **paranoia**. This is where the sufferer sees personal attack around every corner, literal or metaphoric, where there is a delusional belief in some sort of persecution, and where the outcome is going to make the sufferer much worse off in some way.

Irrational jealousy is an example. Let's take a happily married young man who is perceived by a paranoid husband to be making sexual advances on his plain and elderly wife – an unlikely eventuality at any time. But the paranoid husband would be convinced he would be abandoned by his wife (replicating his mother leaving home when he was a child of six), witnessing the friendly meeting between four adults as the opening scene to disaster – for him.

In that case, it is possible the elderly wife could take the subsequent jealous row as flattering to her vanity: he must love her so much he is terrified of losing her. And she takes what was a pleasant peck on the cheek and a welcome hug as a sure sign she is desirable to the young man. We have then a case of collusive folie à deux where, paradoxically, paranoia can be seen as no real problem in a relationship – unless the disorder intensifies, in tandem with other irrational anxieties, and then she might persuade her troubled husband to go into therapy.

But reparation work is difficult. It often seems that no amount of cognitive recognition of where the disorder has sprung from (such as childhood abandonment) can alter the fixed mindset presented. Practitioners hear too many times one partner argue fiercely that such-and-such really did happen, that so-and-so really is out to get them, and so on. Patience and a sensitive understanding of the spouse's rigid beliefs is often the only therapeutic balm to be usefully applied to the troubled victim of paranoia. Even when the therapist has gone straight to the core of the original trauma causing the condition, there is little more to be done when irrational fear has penetrated so deeply into the psyche. As we already know, the unconscious world holds the key – but turning it effectively can sometimes prove impossible.

People with **phobias** have such a wide field into which to pour their anxiety it is possibly even harder for their partner to cope. Phobias can be triggered by a hundred and one unconscious memories, meaningless to an observer but full of impact for the sufferer. Feathers, vegetables, creatures, illness, blood, shadows, the dark, crowded public places, boats, vomit, supermarkets, lifts, escalators, hair dye – the list could go on. As clinical psychologist Roger Baker says in *Understanding Panic Attacks and Overcoming Fear*: 'In the whole area of emotional difficulties there is nowhere that the haunting phrase "destroyed by lack of knowledge" applies more than in panic attacks.' He concludes his book with these words:

> There is much suffering involved in panic; the panic sufferer's life revolves around panic and fear. It is possible to overcome this and return from that terrifying orbit around fear to being able to concentrate on normal everyday life, but when this happens the person will have some catching up to do. The years of concentration on panic often means the sufferer has missed out on so many of the ordinary things in life. Fortunately their problem does not permanently damage their mental faculties which are untouched through the worst panic attack experience. Concentration, memory, feeling at ease – none of this is permanently lost, only temporarily suppressed by fear, and all this can return again.
>
> (1995: 131)

Panic attacks can hit the sufferer at any time of the day or night. They manifest in many kinds of symptoms, from a racing heart, nausea, feeling depersonalized (unreal), dizziness, chest pain, dry mouth, needing to rush to a lavatory to empty bowels or bladder, sweating, trembling and a dread that something terribly wrong is about to happen, such as a heart attack or stroke.

One woman client I worked with told me she always heard a voice in her head at such times saying, 'I'm going to die, I'm going to die!' Interestingly, during therapy she mentioned once that her father 50 years earlier (recently returned from war service with chest injuries) would say exactly that when he struggled for breath – yet she had never before realized the significance of that childhood memory and its legacy for the little daughter who listened.

This client also had difficulty swallowing. Medically diagnosed as *globus hystericus,* the condition is caused by a tightening of the throat muscles brought on by heightened anxiety. She was unable to eat a meal in a restaurant; she could seldom enjoy eating with her own family, preferring to mash up potatoes and protein with a sauce or gravy and take her plateful to another room. The toll on her family in their adult years, celebrating anniversaries and holidays together, was considerable, as might be imagined. But with a strong commitment to therapy, in time her growing understanding of the reasons behind her panic attacks and swallowing problem eased to the point of being able to share in special festivities and to eat meals with her husband at home normally.

I once worked with a pregnant client who, the week she learned she was carrying a child and knowing the foetus required proper nourishment, discovered she could face eating normally and without a moment's difficulty swallowing. Within a few days of her giving birth eight months later to a healthy boy, she unconsciously reverted to the anxiety condition and failed to swallow any food other than mashed potato and (squashed) baked beans. Asked her thoughts on this, she offered, 'I'm not important – but during the pregnancy I was important because I had a baby to feed inside me.' This young mother had sadly been made to feel worthless in her own childhood, with warring parents and a preferred elder sister. It is not difficult to imagine how her low self-esteem unconsciously caused a tightening of throat muscles, refusing to permit nutritious food into serving her body alone. By now, her mother was thrilled with her baby grandson and attentive and loving to her daughter, but the childhood blueprint had been laid down irrevocably – she still believed she was worthless.

Sadly, therapy in her case did not help. Both women clients knew their eating behaviour was irrational. But because they prepared the food in the household, providing meals for their families, they each believed their choice to eat alone in the kitchen was a right that should be respected, little realizing the effect that isolating themselves had upon their husbands and children. For the older woman, her problem improved dramatically once she accepted that her covert activity created divisiveness. Slowly, she learned to eat meals with the family. She took small quantities at first; then as her anxiety lessened that she would choke (remembered childhood fear from a restaurant episode) she relaxed and could join in the domestic scene.

CASE STUDY
Tale of the teeth

Before we conclude the subject of distressing unconscious impact upon our conscious minds I shall turn to the story of the man who found teeth distressing. Teeth as they chewed on strawberries, nuts or anything that made sounds more noticeable. My client and his wife had lived together for nearly 20 years, comfortable in each other's company. However, a personal crisis in his life (unexpected retirement) had somehow raised sediment from the ocean bed of his psyche, stirred up deposits of childhood experience that he had forgotten, or at any rate dismissed as unimportant. The only signs hitherto noticed by his wife that he had an issue with teeth had been years before when he asked her not to tap her teeth, say with a pencil or fingernail, or draw attention to them in any other way.

One afternoon, she announced she was going to make a tomato sandwich for tea, offering him one too. Declining, he went away for an unusually long time before joining her to drink his tea, only to realize she was still munching. He made an excuse and walked away on some supposed errand. He repeated this a second time. Puzzled, she asked him why he was behaving like this, obviously finding her eating suddenly unacceptable. In therapy, he told me:

> 66 I hadn't the faintest idea why I wanted to be away from my wife while she ate her sandwich. All I know is that I found it almost unbearable – the prospect of years ahead having to eat apart loomed and I felt desperate. It was clearly not her fault this unexpected aversion had occurred. I must get to the bottom of it – this is just crazy, after 20 years of easy-going mealtimes. What's happening to me?
>
> (personal communication) 99

Over the next few weeks we explored his childhood. With a largely absent father, interested only in his business, and a cold-hearted mother who favoured his younger twin brothers because they got noticed in the street and admired for their beautiful blonde curls, my client looked back over a bleak early start to life. But the teeth? We wondered about a lack of smiling at him, about the possibility of her ever snarling with anger, showing her teeth like fangs (as a small boy, he might have interpreted her temper as an attacking dog, bent on destroying him). But we had to wait for the answer. Then suddenly he remembered:

> 66 Mother went to the dentist and had all her teeth out, when it was the fashion to have false ones. She told me, however, that as a big baby born in the war years I had drained her of all her calcium, so her teeth went bad. It was my fault she'd lost her teeth, she said. That was so unfair. I didn't deliberately take her calcium – I was only a baby. The injustice of it! Where was consideration of my feelings? Where was her understanding, her sensitivity? No wonder I've had a thing about unfairness all my life – but until now I had never realized why.
>
> (personal communication) 99

If we consider the significance of the mother's thoughtless (and possibly punitive) remark to her little son, we see her jibe betrayed all that a mother should represent: giving the best start, the best nourishment she can for her baby's sake. To show later a resentment that her first born had taken more than his birthright, to her detriment as if he had been greedy and uncaring, flags up a pathology on her part where we might guess she too had been thoughtlessly treated as a child and thought nothing about giving out what she herself had been forced to take. Whatever the cause, her wounding remark was buried deep into the boy's unconscious only to surface decades later first as a quirky dislike of teeth tapping; and then into full-blown revulsion about chewing.

It could be argued that the real issue – though triggered by noisy munching – is about nourishment. Someone else is taking in natural nourishment with the tomato sandwich episode, permitted to relish it without constraint. Could that not remind the little boy of the unfairness meted out to him? In later therapy sessions we worked on his struggle with the current situation in his life, where his retirement had failed to deliver nourishment emotionally, where it seemed so unfair he had lost unexpectedly the employment which had fed so well his sense of self-esteem. All the components in his story began to make sense. And so now he too (like his mother before him) was being punitive to the innocent wife, enjoying her tea-time sandwich in the identical way she had eaten sandwiches all their time together. We have here yet another illustration of the core of a person's current distress having a direct link with the distant past; one requiring psychological excavation work to dislodge it.

My client took only a few more weeks to integrate his new awareness into his conscious mind and – whenever his wife crunched nuts or grapes a tad noisily – he would check his reactive inner response and remind himself of the reason behind it. Gradually, the problem went away. But, as he said, 'These are reflex actions which will take a bit more time to be absorbed into my adult mindset.'

He found a job where workmates valued him and deliberately searched out new interests. Instead of being angry, and projecting negative mother on to his wife, he began to understand that the past could no longer hurt him, that he alone was responsible for taking care of the 'baby within' and that he could find nurturing in his relationships (his wife, children, friends and grand-children) and provide nourishment for his self-esteem in seeking work where he was appreciated.

Summary

Fear lies behind most normal neurotic conditions, as we have seen. Existential fear, fear of humiliation, loss in all its guises, dread disease, confrontation, insects, climbing on buses, change, holidays. It seems that there is no pattern to the various disorders that beset us, and that where one child can cope, another cannot, with resulting emotional trauma to last a lifetime.

Where partners are concerned we must look for the possibility of compatibility (such as the schizoid/hysteric pairing) proving the healing agent for change, once each person has understood the backdrop to the presenting problem. In counselling or therapy, the practitioner needs to be aware of childhood difficulties influencing the present crisis. Getting to the core of each partner's early wounds will inevitably shed more light on the echoes affecting the emotional imbalances now.

In earlier discussion, we see how a gap of decades can lie behind a sudden aversion or disharmony between a couple. The task is to pinpoint the triggers going on in their life currently: what's happened to resonate with hurt from way back? It is important to explore with each client where there seems to be the most 'energy' (or charge) to any given question, or memory offered. One of the chief difficulties facing the practitioner, working with a couple in which fear, obsessions, splitting off, hysterical response or stubborn blocking is central to the session, is in finding a way to help them understand the driving force behind their behaviour. The therapist must be prepared to wait patiently for 'the penny to drop', and for a delay while the other partner can grasp the same revelation.

Not all couples share a sense of goodwill and commitment to change: never underestimate the power of collusion. One partner might enjoy colluding with his or her mate's particular problem – there can be a pay-off in living with someone afflicted with obsessive fear. A pay-off such as being depended upon, being needed, feeling free to expect certain bonuses for their ongoing consideration. I have known of husbands 'earning' rewards in the shape of new motor cycles, rugby supporters' tours, expensive designer clothes – all willingly conceded by grateful wives because they themselves were confined to their homes.

If such collusion works, no one need question it. But a practitioner should keep a wary eye on these domestic deals: a couple could unwittingly be storing up material for later problems of rage and abandonment. Awareness of what they are agreeing to is crucial. It is the therapist's job to ensure that an understanding of the whole picture completes their work together.

In the next chapter, we look at the problems encountered by people in relationships where disorders of a different kind – or tragic difficulties intervene – which affect their emotional well-being together.

5 Asperger and other relationships in trouble

Living with someone with Asperger's Syndrome (AS) can be infuriating and confusing. They find themselves as if sharing a life with a person from a different planet, certainly a different culture. Because there is a similarity in the diagnosed Asperger client to how a schizoid person presents, this parallel can often seem difficult to disentangle. An apparent lack of empathy and inability to 'read' emotional situations can apply to both; and will manifest as splitting off, hard to pinpoint if it is fear (schizoid) driving it, or a brain abnormality (Asperger's).

Research has not yet (at the time of writing) shown any clear indication as to what causes the syndrome, although as Tony Attwood says in his book *Asperger's Syndrome: A Guide For Parents and Professionals:* 'There is increasing evidence to suggest the frontal and temporal lobes of the brain are dysfunctional. This has been suggested by the results of studies using a range of neuropsychological tests and brain imaging techniques' (1998: 143). He goes on to suggest that the incidence of obstetric abnormalities is high, whether in pre-, peri- or post-natal crises, and that brain damage may cause or at least affect the degree of expression of a condition already genetically predisposed. There is also a possibility of viral infection in early infancy to account for it.

CASE STUDY
Living with Asperger's Syndrome

Chloe, mother of three children, did not experience any difficulties, however, around the birth of her daughter Lucy, who was diagnosed with Asperger's Syndrome when a little girl at primary school. Although Lucy's father has not been diagnosed, Chloe is convinced that the condition was inherited from him. Ten years living with this unusual man – 'kind, laid-back, bizarre' – finally proved to her she had chosen a husband with no common sense:

> 66 I would ask him to go to the shops for cucumber and cheese and he'd come back with nothing, or biscuits and a tin of baked beans. He didn't seem to register what is being said. He once took our toddler daughter out for the day without putting any shoes on her feet. On another occasion, she had covered herself all over with cream, smeared on her face, dress, hair and hands, and he was completely unaware.
>
> I could be crying, distraught about something and making sobbing noises but he would come into the room and turn on the television, look at me and then ask what were we going to have for tea. It was exhausting living with him. I had to take all the responsibility and do everything to ensure we as a family got out of the house on time. When I think back, I saw him at first as a kind 'yes' man, who'd avoid confrontation and keep saying 'Oh, sorry love' if I got upset, but he was incapable of reading the true situation and dealing with it.
>
> (personal communication) 99

Chloe discovered she was pregnant with their third child. After a few months into the pregnancy her husband walked out one day with no explanation. He answered her telephone calls, promising he would be home that evening and that 'It's going to be all right', then not arrive. This went on for the next few months, until shortly before she was due to give birth Chloe tracked him down to his new place of work – as a policeman. The police station superintendent had no idea he was a married man with two daughters and a baby due and sent him home to Chloe. He did not arrive and was duly signed off by the superintendent as sick, classified as a missing person.

> 66 I finally tracked him down by hiding behind a hedge outside a supermarket and told him he had to face the fact he'd got a family and the girls would need him to look after them when I had the baby. He texted me every day – hundreds, I've kept them – and then one day did come home, and told the girls he'd been away training to be a policeman. The girls laid a place for him at the table every day after, sitting at the window waiting for him. He never came and we were all heartbroken. After my son was born (we did get a brief visit then), he continued his bizarre behaviour until I told him I was going to divorce him.
>
> (personal communication) 99

When highly intelligent Lucy was showing problems at school, Chloe sought help for her, certain that her daughter had inherited a condition of some sort. Again, the unawareness and the unseeing eye. Lucy would call out to her mother, 'I can't find my shoes, Mummy, where are they?' only to be told they were there by her feet. Choosing a new beaker in a busy shop became a nightmare outing for both mother and child when Lucy agonized over the colour. Did she like the blue one or the green? As soon as a decision had been made, she would burst into tears and beg for the other instead. Finally (after many repetitions) the homecoming with a new beaker was marred by her little girl crying for the next three hours about bringing home 'the wrong colour'.

People with AS are usually told theirs is a condition which cannot be cured. But there is some evidence to show that its affects can be modified, with the help of a sympathetic parent or partner. Where they understand the diffi- culties, as did Chloe with both husband and daughter struggling with the condition, they can encourage their family member to perform social rituals so that their unusual behaviour will be disguised.

One client learned to ask his wife to be the first to make contacts in new situations like parties, introducing her husband who would then take it as his cue to offer his hand to shake, while making the (learned) pleasantries to ease the initial shy start. She would prime him with conversational topics likely to arise and keep a watchful eye to steer him away if an emotionally confusing scene should crop up where, say, someone might announce a sad death. Someone with AS would probably have no idea what best to say next. Their world may not hold an ability to empathize with the bereaved and danger could then lurk in them making an unaware, inappropriate remark.

Not as they seem

Social skills are hard for the Asperger sufferer. Gisela Slater-Walker, who married Chris not knowing he suffered from the syndrome (diagnosed six years later), describes in their jointly written *An Asperger Marriage*: 'For many women (Asperger Syndrome is much more common in men than women), the diagnosis . . . has followed years of unhappiness in which their husband's behaviour had been eccentric to say the least and, in many cases, the marriage had been irreparably damaged' (2002: 14). She goes on to say:

> 66 The most difficult thing about Asperger Syndrome, from my perspective, is that it is always easy to mistake autistic behav- iour from such an able person as being deliberately unso- ciable or manipulative, when almost invariably it is not. I can understand why people not on the spectrum find this inability to communicate so difficult to understand. Chris's

> hearing is excellent; he has a very good musical ear and is multilingual. . . . Yet, he finds it painfully difficult to under-stand other people in a setting where there is a lot of back-ground noise, and cups his hand around his ear to try to help concentrate on the one voice. He finds it hard to follow more than one conversation at a time, though his command of the English language is apparently perfect, to the point where he cannot help correcting others.
>
> (2002: 84–5) **99**

Relationships like theirs need a good communicator within the partnership, obviously not the AS person. The Slater-Walkers found that in the early days of getting to know one another making the effort to communicate together was comparatively easy. 'But when communication becomes an essential rather than a nicety, for example, to sort out misunderstandings, or provide sympathy, then this is where relationships can suffer.'

The couple found emailing one another useful, even when they might both be in the same house and not at their respective workplaces. Email allows Chris to say how he feels as he has more time to collect his thoughts and express them without any external pressure. The 'instant message' facilities on the internet have been a boon for them:

> **66** This has allowed us to have some fruitful and, from Chris, some very witty exchanges. I have really enjoyed these, and though Chris may be 25 miles away, I can feel closer to him than when he is in the same room. . . . It may be the physical distance between us which means that all he has to deal with in the exchange is the words I have written, totally uncom-plicated by any non-verbal communication that can be more complex for him to understand – such as anger or irrita-tion. . . . The fact that there is time to think between exchanges without any pressure to respond is helpful to Chris as well. It seems easier for him to express himself too and there is less possibility of being misunderstood because the tone of his voice does not match his words.
>
> (2002: 86) **99**

Sexual compatibility for the Slater-Walkers proved an unexpected bonus. Anecdotal evidence suggests there can be some difficulties where one partner has Asperger's Syndrome, for sensory issues and feelings of isolation in the non-spectrum partner can be the cause of deep unhappiness. Clinical psychol-ogist Tony Attwood recalls the husband of a client with AS complaining his wife 'was too cold and aloof, and that when he was showing affection it was "like hugging a plank of wood".' Attwood adds:

" The partners may need counselling on each other's background and perspective. One could describe the relationship as similar to a marriage between two people from very different cultures, unaware of the conventions and expectations of the other partner. They unwittingly step on each other's toes. The author often uses the analogy of a person from a different culture to explain the problems experienced by the person with Asperger's Syndrome and the people they meet.

Certainly in the early courtship days parents may have to provide some explanations to boyfriends or girlfriends who are confused as to why the person is so different regarding physical intimacy and rarely uses the words and gestures of love and affection. This may also be relevant for families and younger children.

(1998: 167) "

When Gisela Slater-Walker discovered she was pregnant, she found to her delight that Chris was fascinated by the pregnancy and 'his sense of wonder at the process was uplifting. He liked to feel the baby kicking and wanted to know how it felt to be pregnant. He would look at the "lump" and I never had any sense of him finding me unattractive; in fact, it was quite the opposite, he still made me feel very feminine right through the pregnancy' (2002: 123).

Alcohol and depression

CASE STUDY
Fatherhood and AS

Not all parents are so fortunate. I once worked with a couple where both pregnancies were viewed by the forthcoming father as depressing. An AS sufferer himself, remembering the lonely and isolated childhood he had experienced not being understood either by his parents or his peers, David viewed the future for any offspring of his with dispiriting gloom. His usually cheerful wife, Kiera, looked back on the arrival of their two sons, six and four years earlier, with sadness. David had taken to drinking steadily every evening he returned home from work as a salesman.

At first he explained he had to unwind because of the stress at work. Then he blamed his drinking on being woken up at all hours when Kiera breastfed her child, expecting him at least to change nappies occasionally to help her rest. There would be new reasons as the years went by to convince him of the need to drink. David broke down during one session in therapy and said, 'I can't stand it. The strain of having children is beyond my capability. The elder boy has diagnosed Asperger's, and it now looks likely little Fred has the condition. The irony is,' he added, 'I understand what they are and what they will go through in life, but it is as if I am looking at my sons from the outside, appalled at the responsibility in caring for them. No wonder I turn to alcohol. But I do realize it can't go on like this much longer.'

He and his wife continued in therapy together for a few more months. We had spent the time quite usefully, exploring the actual episodes behind David's childhood which caused him grief, undoubtedly leading to serious depression during his adolescence, and now reactivated by the arrival of his sons. He loved the boys deeply, but he found domestic life stressful. As he said, he understood the boys' unusual behaviour patterns, but cognition did not rule out his impatience. Kiera was an instinctive mother, spending hours and hours attending to her children's needs and, of course, sometimes to the detriment of their own relationship.

'So what if Kiera hasn't found the time to tidy up the toy cupboard?' I wondered, aloud. 'Could you not feel it time better spent when instead she plays and draws pictures with the boys if they want her company? Kiera has told us here that she stays up until after midnight most evenings just trying to catch up with housework and chores. Perhaps you feel a bit neglected, David? Where's special time for you? Where's special time for Kiera? It seems to me she's knocking herself out trying to be a good mother, wife and specialist carer for Fred and Joe: you both need a break!'

My comment was greeted with raised eyebrows: how *could* I suggest them taking a short holiday away from the boys? Even though, yes, one or the other grandparents would be glad to cooperate (and could manage the challenge), David and Kiera seemed to think leaving their children for a few days was out of the question; it was not up for discussion, impossible to contemplate. Now this seemed a pity. There was real danger in crises looming ahead, either through drink-related problems or emotional breakdown, or both. Taking stock now and planning some rest together would recharge their relationship and provide energy and determination to carry on as a family.

A self-destruct cloud seemed to hang over them as we sat in the room. My guess was that David was too deeply depressed to imagine the benefit of taking time out of parenthood; that at some level he paradoxically relished his trapped state, as he perceived it: it fed his misery in a circular round of stress, drink, sleep, stress. Also that Kiera was so exhausted in her role as carer of at least two males with Asperger's Syndrome, she could only see herself function on a one-day-at-a-time basis, blinkered by tiredness and so angry with her husband for opting out of sharing the work, she actually preferred domestic routine to a holiday alone with him.

It came as no surprise the following week when Kiera announced that the childminder who collected the boys from school (so that they could come to therapy) had said she could no longer do the job. Living as they did in a remote village two miles from the primary school, there seemed no solution but to stop their therapy. Going deeper into the unconscious world can be daunting for some; and for David and Kiera they were overwhelmed, both by unconscious and (appropriate) conscious concerns.

Bolshie teenager

The final case to discuss in this section concerns another kind of problem experienced by the partner of a person suffering with Asperger's Syndrome.

Annie is convinced her computer technician husband should be diagnosed as having the syndrome because Jeremy matches up to most of the pointers she has read about. However, at 50 years old he is not likely to be encouraged to seek intervention, she believes, and so has to struggle with the fall-out from his AS symptoms without the comforting label to explain them. Jeremy at times seems, despite his age and professional competence, like a 'bolshie, stubborn 13 year old'. He disappears to the local pub for four hours on a Sunday, tying up their dog outside, regardless of the temperature. Alcohol is a constant source of comfort to him, needing as he does casual company to assuage his loneliness. Annie goes on:

> The future is daunting for me. Even though Jeremy has not been diagnosed, without question in my mind he has Asperger's Syndrome, and he responds well to the offered strategies I've discovered through my reading, to help overcome his difficulties. So much so, actually, I think I've created a monster! When we met he was terribly under-confident, so I would praise him to build up his confidence. But by teaching him to speak out, it seemed to give him licence to be rude in public. We were at a checkout in a supermarket recently and Jeremy said loudly, 'Oh no! We've got Shit Brains at this till, let's move to another checkout.' I was mortified. Then, at the chemist, he said to a young girl assistant, 'This is your first day here, isn't it?' She looked really offended. We'd only just come from another shop where an assistant had apologized for her slow speed and said this was her first day at the job. AS people take things so literally, they can't understand nuances: so for Jeremy, a new job means everyone gets flustered on their first day.
>
> (personal communication)

An interesting observation from Attwood comes via Digby Tantam, who researched at considerable length and depth into the condition discussed in the various cases above, and wrote a definitive paper for *The British Journal of Psychiatry*. Referring to this, Attwood comments at the end of his own book:

> 66 Digby Tantam has used the term 'lifelong eccentricity', to describe the long-term outcome of individuals with Asperger's Syndrome (1988). The term eccentricity is not used in a derogatory sense. In this author's opinion, they are a bright thread in the rich tapestry of life. Our civilisation would be extremely dull and sterile if we did not have and treasure people with Asperger's Syndrome.
>
> (1998: 185) 99

When tragedy strikes

After decades of happiness together, couples who have never experienced relationship difficulties such as those described in the preceding text, can be doubly hard hit when a health crisis occurs. Any one major illness is difficult to come to terms with, but all are certain to shatter domestic security, the comfort of day-to-day routine for partners who long ago had learned to depend upon their delight in each other: not to take their relationship for granted, but to regard their life as the solid rock on which that relationship flourished, unequivocally safe.

For Alan (mentioned in Chapter 1) that solid rock shook when a consultant diagnosed Alzheimer's Disease in his beloved wife Hilary. For some time previously Hilary had been showing signs of difficulty in coping with driving, shopping, remembering things. One day, after agreeing to meet up after various errands in town, Alan waited for two hours until he saw Hilary walking past without recognizing him. He grabbed her arm, both of them upset and angry.

> 66 She went quiet then, and not long after that day she said she ought to see our doctor who in turn referred her to a psychiatrist. That led to continuous interviews, testings – nine months' process which was (in the National Health Service system) frankly horrendous, before we had the diagnosis. Coping with her then at our house over the next two years was physically very hard. Eventually, our grown-up children and I decided she should go into a home. Hilary had developed loose bowels, so we couldn't trust not being near the bathroom. If we tried going

for a little walk, her legs might suddenly collapse and I would have to carry her home.

Yet all the way through, she and I have kept up contact at an intuitive level. We have entered a very strange territory which I guess some people would call spiritual territory, where it doesn't occur to me remotely that however bad she gets it will be any less than that.

My sorrow for her, to see her hacked down like a tree remorselessly [by the disease], that quite broke my heart. One of the worst moments I remember was when friends said 'You've got to look after yourself' after Hilary had been admitted to the home, and when nurses said 'Cheer up!' I wanted to say 'Fuck off!', I was so angry. I don't want to use strategies, I live my anger. It feels more honest, even when it hurts so much sometimes, but I would rather hurt than pretend.

(personal communication) **"**

On his twice-daily visits to see Hilary, Alan would frequently say to her 'You will never know how much I love you', holding her hand and – after nine long months of silence – not expecting a response beyond her squeezing his hand back. Then one day she spoke the words 'I love you' clearly. Hearing is the last faculty to go with Alzheimer patients, and Alan takes comfort from the fact that Hilary could understand what he had talked to her about during his visits. He asked for forgiveness if he should ever have hurt her in their long life together; he talked to her as if carrying on a conversation. If tears filled her eyes, it seemed to help Hilary when Alan interpreted: 'You feel sad.'

Theirs is a moving story and illustrates how a relationship can survive the most terrible difficulties and yet nourish both partners despite those difficulties. Alan's account speaks without words of the hidden richness their tragedy wove for them spiritually through Hilary's illness, one which removed her from their normal life yet continued the strength of its intimacy; as Alan believes, in a strange territory where the setting and disability held no significance.

How others cope

Living with illness, where the patient returns from hospital after treatment but might then need either convalescence or indefinite care at home, is obviously traumatic. Both partners, whether carer or patient, will be thrown into a vortex of emotional turmoil, neither able to hold the new situation easily or take the crisis in their stride. Resentment, dependency, exhaustion and despair will all too easily slide into their lives now, however much they faced the sudden blow of illness or accident with stoicism.

How often do we hear cancer patients declare resolutely 'We'll fight this!' only to watch them later sink into lethargy; or stroke victims at first speaking optimistically about driving and walking again, realizing much later that neither would be possible. For women who have had a hysterectomy, or a single or double mastectomy, the turmoil they may experience leaving hospital for home may not focus on their fears of a poor prognosis, but on their anxiety that they will still be attractive to their partner. Sensitive issues like this will need sensitive counselling. It is unlikely to serve the anxious ex-patient by rushing in to reassure them that of course their husband will find them as desirable as ever. They may not. In this scenario, grief will be presented sooner or later in the therapy room; the couple have lost their sexual pleasure in each other and the wife is in despair. The practitioner will need to sit with her, contain her depression and anger ('Is it my fault I got cancer?') and wait until she slowly comes to terms with the new situation.

As Dennis Brown and Jonathan Pedder say in *Introduction to Psychotherapy*, there are times when the most that a therapist can do is just be there, tolerating anxiety and uncertainty: 'surviving as a reliable concerned person (perhaps also surviving the patient's hostility and demands for immediate action and gratification) until such time as things become clearer and understanding is finally reached' (1979: 86–7).

And what of the partners involved? For some, their life will be indefinitely changed, whether this involves their sexual activity, socializing or just plain domestic routine. For others, that change might not prove so drastic, perhaps because they have home help, or the patient can manage well on their own during the day. Lives are not always upturned, although priority must be given to the patient's best interests. If there are young children in the house, provision has to be made to see their own lives are disrupted as little as possible: chatting over their day with the invalid parent, homework, sharing television viewing together and preferably also meals.

For couples whose sexual life has been an important part of their relationship, the sudden disappearance of libido or ability after illness or accident is likely to be a great loss. For the healthy partner, it will mean an enforced time of frustration. Some may eventually seek release elsewhere, often haunted by guilt even when they have been encouraged to do so by the sick spouse. Counselling such cases needs delicate probing. Does their husband (or wife) really know, or is it implicit that outside sexual relationships are to be tolerated? Often a partner will want to believe they have been given licence, yet feel guilty in taking it anyway, probably without checking first with the invalid.

It is by no means straightforward but a delicate situation requiring delicate negotiation. In the therapy room, it may be necessary to draw out the issue from the carer, who could be reluctant to risk appearing selfish against the backdrop of disease or invalidism. Better to discuss their needs and fears, however, in the safe holding of the therapy room than that they keep secret their private thoughts until they erupt at home, perhaps causing far more distress.

Communication is always to be encouraged in such situations. However, where the patient at home is considered to be in a vulnerable state, unlikely to be clear about their true thoughts, then the client should be aware that he or she may have to make adult decisions on their own, choosing a course of action as a grown up rather than take the infantile position: 'Mummy/Daddy says I can, so I will.' If a couple have arrived nonetheless at agreement about lovers, then consideration will need to be given to subsequent feelings of jealousy, or dread that an external relationship might tempt the able-bodied partner away.

Sexual needs may not come into the equation at all. The couple at home may find themselves content to put their sexual life behind them, or both partners discover an unexpected benefit paradoxically resulting from illness in that they are relieved of a not-so-satisfactory sexual obligation to one another. There can be other bonuses too. One client, married to a woman with myalgic encephalopathy (ME) or chronic fatigue syndrome, reluctantly admitted he liked the social freedom her predicament gave him.

Finding a compromise

As a reward for looking after her so well each evening when he returned home from work, his wife suggested he play golf frequently with his men friends, and even encouraged him to make up a four to fly abroad to play on foreign golf courses. Somehow, they had found a compromise which worked for them; a form of collusive practice which kept man and wife in a reciprocal arrangement of mutual benefit. In return for her gesture, he gave her what she needed – his devotion, morning and night – and she gave him permission to go out to play with his friends. Yes, this was a mother and son relationship and not one (as this chapter's title suggests) actually in trouble. It might even seem the opposite, given the respective satisfaction with the status quo. Neither the client nor his *puella* wife (described in Chapter 3) unconsciously wished to grow up. Having an indulgent 'mother' suited the *puer* 'boy'. Materially successful, he could afford not only his outdoor games but to pay for overnight carers when he was away from home on his pleasure trips. Unfortunately, this collusive practice carried a stagnant quality about it, where neither partner could grow in psychological maturity.

People do recover from ME, but this woman had taken permanently to her bed over a considerable number of years, unconsciously choosing the safety of her bedroom for fear of the challenge in trying to return to health and outside responsibilities. It is not being suggested that this condition, or any other disabling illness, has a neurotic root cause. But as the debate continues over chronic fatigue syndrome (psychological or viral?) it does provide a useful example of the possibility of psychosomatic origin, however. Brown and Pedder argue that people may become ill and present problems to a potential helper, such as a doctor, when in unbearable conflict with unacceptable and often unconscious aspects of themselves or their relationships (a central theme in previous chapters here). They offer:

> 66 The patient's need for symptoms and defences has to be explored, understood, and *worked through* – repeatedly experienced and resolved – before he can give up what has been called the *primary gain*: that is the advantage in terms of immediate freedom from emotional discomfort. If they are prolonged, as with any disability, the sufferer may learn to make the best of his neurotic symptoms and defences. They come to have a social function, maintaining certain roles and relationships which might bring advantages; for example, sympathetic consideration may be gained, along with covert revenge for its having been previously withheld. In some families it is difficult to gain attention, and illness may be the only means of being noticed as being a person with special needs.
>
> (1979: 85) 99

This topic, though of great importance in the wider field of mental health, is not one which can be pursued here. Among many excellent publications in this genre, readers interested in exploring further how our thinking affects our bodies may like to read: J.R. Millenson (1982) *Mind Matters: Psychological Medicine in Holistic Practice*; L.Temoshok and H. Dreher (1992) *The Type C Connection: The Behavioral Links to Cancer and Your Health*; P. Pietroni (1986) *Holistic Living*.

Summary

When illness or brain dysfunction affect a couple there are difficulties thrown up as unpredictable as they are painful. Whether it be a major illness – cancer, stroke, heart attack – or of a less threatening kind, disease becomes the centre of a family's life. Partners, children, relatives are all drawn into the intense drama playing itself out, and inevitably emotional crises will result. Lives will be turned upside down. Diagnosis almost always proves a watershed: everyone involved has something to 'hold on to', a label which explains much and helps adjustment.

But if there is no diagnosis, as in the case of some Asperger's Syndrome men and women (particularly if middle-aged who have managed to function out in the world comparatively normally), the difficulties encountered in intimate relationship can be bewildering. Partners can make little sense of what they see as bizarre behaviour and – worse – they cannot make their loved one understand their frustration.

Sometimes a couple will present for therapy to sort out their problems with a third party, whose job it is to try to understand both sides of the predicament. As we have seen before, carefully explaining the likely sources for disagreement and manageable strategies for AS sufferers can work well. Each person will need to respect the special requirements involved. The AS partner might, for example, find partner-to-partner communication easier sometimes via email, because he or she can take time to assimilate the words more easily in a turbulent situation.

When a client comes for counselling or therapy on their own to discuss illness at home, their greatest need will be for a safe, holding environment where they feel free to pour out their grief, fears, guilt, or indeed relief. It is not unknown for one partner secretly to welcome the breakdown in health of their mate, for it might mean a new freedom they had long wanted. (This does not refer to the Alzheimer case study above.) The therapist must be prepared for any confession and to go with the revelations without judgement, helping their client to be aware of the implications of their feelings, to be honest with themselves and to take responsibility for what they do or do not do.

The next chapter concerns other difficulties encountered, where flawed thinking, borderline psychosis and inherited belief systems can cause great emotional damage, though more subtle than in the previous, more obviously defined cases.

6 Inherited faulty thinking, toxic belief systems

Lack of nurturing throughout generations can have dire consequences. Faulty thinking on the part of one or both parents, inherited of course from their own parents (who in turn probably received similar insensitive treatment), can and does pass down the line unchallenged. Who was there, after all, to do the challenging? A young child only knows about what goes on in their home, they have no other point of reference.

If two little sisters are left eating crisps outside the pub in the dark while their Mum and Dad drink heavily for hours, it is likely they will grow into women who do not consider the emotional welfare of their own children. If the son of a steelworker knows only poverty, brutal language and to avoid his sick, angry father when he is in a rage, then he will grow up unable to show affection to his offspring.

When a daughter is constantly told by her anxious mother 'If I drop dead in the street when we're out, then you're to go to a nice lady and tell her where you live' she will go into adulthood terrified herself of dropping dead in the street. This particular woman, Pat, was as a child of three sent away to Scotland to stay (inexplicably) with her grandparents, only to learn when she was finally collected three months later that she now had a baby brother. The shock of abandonment and sense of rejection stayed with her for life, as did the fear of sudden death. But to prove to herself she was strong enough to look after her vulnerable mother over the following years, Pat would go to find broken glass in the dustbin to cut her hand and endure the pain. A counsellor now, Pat insists to this day that her only motivation was to discover how much she could cope with – a badly cut finger was not meant to curry sympathy. She knew she was unlikely to get it. Her practice was to keep testing herself that she was robust enough to look after her mother. As David Edwards and Michael Jacobs point out in *Conscious and Unconscious*, by age three children 'can already guide their own behaviour by spoken self-instruction, and in due course this self-instruction takes place covertly' (2003: 97).

What the stories here tell us is that above and beyond poor education, poverty, cultural tenets of the day and so on, a fundamental lack of psychological maturity lies behind much of the distress unwittingly meted out to children. We are aware of the accounts of Victorian upbringing, where children (in middle and upper class families) were expected to be silent unless spoken to and would expect to see their parents virtually by appointment. This seeming lack of interest, whatever the class, smacks of a remoteness of affect; attachment needs unmet other than in the wealthier home perhaps, where nannies would provide some form of primary caregiving.

We learn from psychiatrist and psychoanalyst John Bowlby, who formulated the concept of attachment theory and wrote about it extensively in his *Attachment and Loss* series (1969–75), that infants need proximity to an attachment figure in stressful situations; certainly from nine months to three years of age when it reaches its peak. Thus we see the need for a secure base, whether via a caregiver or sensitive mother, to become an essential component in a child's development when he or she starts to move outwards. Each stage in that development may be compromised, as with the careless pub-drinking parents leaving their daughters unattended and lonely on the doorstep. The danger is that a child's emotional life goes no further than the base line.

Fathers and sons

One client inherited emotional illiteracy from his father, whose own father had suffered severe hardship working in Welsh quarries, often unemployed and hungry, unable to feed his large family. The oldest boy was sent away to try to make his own living – it did not matter where or how – and so this 16-year-old lad found himself alone, angry and despairing. He joined the Army as soon as he could, finding the semblance of family in its structure and routine. Eventually he met his wife (also the product of a bleak childhood) and discovered they had conceived a child which neither wanted. Peter recalls:

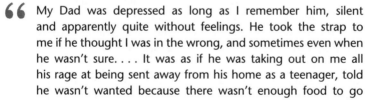

My Dad was depressed as long as I remember him, silent and apparently quite without feelings. He took the strap to me if he thought I was in the wrong, and sometimes even when he wasn't sure. . . . It was as if he was taking out on me all his rage at being sent away from his home as a teenager, told he wasn't wanted because there wasn't enough food to go round.

Of course, that probably wasn't the full story: my grandparents weren't ogres and they were driven with fear about surviving. Their oldest boy stood as good a chance as anyone of making a living somewhere, so they decided they should send him away. He never forgave them. Now, I have difficulty in forgiving my father and mother for withholding love and affection from me as a boy. But what had they to look back on? A wasteland of depression and anxiety in the family home respectively.

(personal communication) 99

In Richard Madeley's autobiography, *Fathers And Sons*, he describes a story of abandonment and betrayal also so painful that it is almost unbelievable. His grandfather, Geoffrey, only ten years old and excitedly expecting to be setting sail next day in 1907 with the rest of his family for a new life in Canada, woke up to find them gone. In return for the price of eight one-way fares, both parents had agreed in secrecy to leave Geoffrey behind to help his uncle at Kiln Farm. He had been told nothing. It would be more than a decade before he would see his parents and six brothers and sisters again.

Geoffrey in due course had children of his own. When his son Christopher was a little boy of four, imaginatively trying to plant a chocolate biscuit outdoors to grow a tree of them, Geoffrey exploded with rage. This was the time of the Great Depression in the 1930s and few luxuries were available. Geoffrey reached for a cane and beat his small son, accusing him of 'wicked waste'. Then, when Richard Madeley was himself only seven, Christopher gave his son a savage beating, repeating such cane punishments over the next few years. Madeley comments in his book: 'I see my father's violent outbreaks towards me as a kind of descent into madness.' One day, Christopher tried to explain his rages by saying he thought they were something to do with his boyhood, much like his own father's, lashing out against his bitter experiences:

66 I think this was probably at the heart of it. And I have supporting evidence; the domino effect of these beatings clicked and tripped its painful way into my own childhood.

But these almost ritualised punishments – the sacred stick broadcasting its mute warning from corner to cupboard; the appointed place of execution (always the parlour where the best furniture was) – were not peculiar to Kiln Farm. They were de rigueur for the day. Most parents still imposed discipline on their children according to the Victorian mantra of 'spare the rod and spoil the child'. Fathers – and mothers too – cheerfully wielded straps, canes, belts, rulers and shoes on their erring sons and daughters and would have been astounded to be told they were child-abusers.

(2009: 64) 99

Attachment patterns

In her book *The Relate Guide To Finding Love*, couples and family counsellor and supervisor Barbara Bloomfield addresses these transgenerational attachment patterns. Acknowledging many people do try to correct the messages they received in their upbringing, creating instead more loving and stable relationships for themselves, she goes on to say:

> But as Relate counsellors who work with many couples with relationship difficulties, we cannot help but frequently see patterns of attachment – both helpful and not so helpful – flowing from grandparents to parents and parents to children, however hard individuals might try not to repeat them.
>
> At moments of stress and crisis these patterns can be especially noticeable as they become the 'default' setting that we fall into when we are under a great deal of pressure. For example, Megan noticed that when people raised their voices, she tended to withdraw and leave the room before any discussion or debate could get going. To hide under the table had been her childhood 'strategy' for dealing with her high-decibel parents, whose frequent and unpredictable arguments had scared her. But, as an adult, the withdrawal strategy was not helping her to grow as an individual because men saw her as a timid woman who shrank from interesting and lively discussions.
>
> (2009: 27–8)

Attachment, as Barbara Bloomfield later explains, is a special emotional relationship involving the exchange of care, comfort and pleasure, a lasting psychological connectedness between human beings. She cites one study she had researched which said that the likelihood of a parent passing on their own attachment style to their offspring is as high as 80 per cent. In an interview with her for this book, I sought her views on those earlier days of our forefathers when the quality of connectedness was so evidently missing. She said:

> Victorians had no way of describing their inner life. Freud didn't begin to percolate into society until the beginning of the twentieth century and then only in the higher echelons. And between the 1900s and the 1950s what could attachment mean? They couldn't go there because they were losing so many of their children: with disease and with wars. Nowadays, most of our

children survive, but our grandparents often lost as many as four or more children, in the Victorian and Edwardian periods. Such loss must have forged a different way of thinking, of relating to their families.

(personal communication) **99**

This attitude, of course, would explain Geoffrey Madeley's parents deserting him overnight on the practical rationale of survival: one able-bodied boy left behind to work the farm for the man who handed his relatives the money to make a new life in Canada. It is hard to understand their reasoning; hard to grasp that a mother could (though surely emotionally torn?) permit such ruthlessness. That the abandonment did cause grievous and lasting suffering is evident from the men's rage towards the next generation.

Poverty was a hugely contributory factor for so many families in the past, where shortage of food was their primary concern. If a child died, then this meant one less mouth to feed; if the man of the household lost work or fell sick, the woman and her children would go hungry or end up in the workhouse. Niceties such as attachment love, safe holding, sensitive listening – what room was there in that environment for such luxuries? The world of talking therapy would have seemed a meaningless set of alien messages from outer space.

Small wonder that in succeeding generations, no longer hungry, working families had little to say to one another other than an extension perhaps of the earlier topics which would have preoccupied them: employment chances, wages, material goods and the best options for security. Coming from such families, young men had learned little of the value of showing affection, of respecting the delight and giftedness of their own children. Sadly, this is why many present-day middle-aged male clients report the dearth of affection shown them by their fathers when they were young. As Alix Pirani points out in her book *The Absent Father*:

66 Fathers vary in the degree to which they can tolerate the disparity between the role they thought they were to adopt and what fathering has turned out to be. . . . The challenge at present is to get the absent father to return: whatever that means in its context. What seems to have happened is that the fathers who have been banished, or have withdrawn themselves, are still in a state of shock, not quite sure what has hit them, trying to avoid feeling the pain, guilt, bewilderment, and vaguely hoping the mothers will sort it out for them. The mothers do their best (by writing books on the subject, for instance) but that isn't enough. The absent father needs to contact his inner Perseus, work through the feelings he probably has about his wife, family, society, and the

Medusa proportions they may have assumed, and go on to use his imagination and all available resources to help restore his sense of himself and his potential as a man and a progenitor.

(1988: 118) **99**

We see their dilemma. Men over the generations learned from their fathers to be silent and undemonstrative, unconsciously teaching their sons to do the same. Showing love and joy in their family was considered unnecessary, if it was considered at all. Shouting at them, strapping them when they were naughty, or merely making jokes at the children's expense would be standard behaviour. And those habits linger on.

For example, one present-day young father entertaining friends in the garden aimed for an appreciative laugh, aware of his six-year-old son playing boisterously nearby. 'Someone get me my gun,' he quipped, 'I've had enough of this noise.' The little boy heard the remark, looked shocked and, of course, stopped his game. He knew he would not get hurt; that was not the point. Real contact with his father was seldom there; he was usually the butt for his father to make an easy joke. Not difficult to guess here the child's already low sense of self, an increasing lack of worth in a family where his idol regularly made unthinking put-down remarks. But this was replicating how the young man himself had been treated as a boy. He knew no other way.

Women's subservient role

Where are the women in all of this? The gender issue was a major schism in the families of the past, where the father 'knew best' and the mother's subservient role typified the prevailing rule for generations. Disempowered, subordinate to her husband, a woman had relatively no voice and was usually dependent for her living on her husband. With no birth control available, she would expect to conceive many pregnancies, and probably lose several too. Other than those from the upper classes, who could afford domestic and nursery help, most women would also find themselves exhausted. Young children would often be looked after by the older children. It is hardly surprising that sibling rivalry, petty jealousies and bullying were rife in those days with only the luckier youngsters finding themselves lovingly cared for, praised and understood by an older sister or brother.

Faulty thinking? It was there in abundance, obscured in part by the mores of the time, but there in the heart of the family, with its prejudices, fear of neighbours' criticism, the need for good presentation, the quest for respectability at all costs and, not least, the dread of the local minister's wrath. Where was the scope for emotional development as present-day therapists would want to encourage?

Living as they did in a culture where 'Thou Shalt Not' was a lifetime creed, it is unsurprising that most young people grew up afraid to step out of line, still in the grip of some form of fear. Paramount now was social survival. The driving force was a quest for good appearance, to be admired and quite possibly envied.

Guilt played – and still does – a huge part in forging some of the faulty thinking that our forebears carried in their psyches; guilt instilled largely by the religion of the day, but also by a stern patriarchal upbringing, linked undoubtedly with the former. As one young client said, 'I was brought up to the sounds of "We love you despite who you are", not unconditional love. That made me view my parents as saints, in that they still could be fond of me even though I clearly wasn't lovable. When my future husband once said to me "I love you because you are you", I wept. No one had ever said that to me before.'

Toxic belief systems such as this appear in different guises. One grandfather overheard his daughter lavishly praising her two-year-old boy and looked appalled. 'Never praise him, he'll get big headed!' he warned, seriously alarmed. This was a man who as a child regularly used to get locked in the cupboard under the stairs for being naughty. Never hearing a word of praise for anything good he might do, naturally he grew up believing that he would make his own child unpopular if she got an inflated idea of herself. Little did he realize that she needed all the encouragement she could get, struggling into adulthood despite the deprivation. She determined therefore to change the pattern with her own child, encouraging at every turn. In therapy, this young woman remembered:

> 66 I would work my socks off at school to get good marks to please him, and bring back the report where I might have been given 99 marks out of 100. My father would pick up the piece of paper and ask me what went wrong with the other mark, why had I missed that question? I don't ever recall him saying 'Well done!' This all came back to me the other day when I had returned home, tired and hungry, only to be bitten by our puppy. Irrationally, I felt like saying to this little dog 'After all I've done for you, working hard to earn the money to feed you and take you for walks, and then you go and *bite* me. It's not fair!' Now you have asked me what that resentful feeling reminds me of, my father springs to mind, of course: I take my frustration at him out on a puppy – ten years too late.
>
> (personal communication) 99

Another toxic belief potentially poisoning family life occurs where children are exposed to faulty thinking inherited from adults apart from their parents. Phrases like 'Be a good boy, or Granny/Grandpa/Auntie won't love you anymore' have all the traumatic conditional implication mentioned above. It is tempting to add here that this admonition is only one step away from the dire warnings in the Christian bible that wrongdoers will be punished.

Client Phillipa was ruefully beginning to understand how much her upbringing in a convent had unconsciously influenced her to set up unhealthy collusive ways in dealing with her family. Driven by 'shoulds and oughts', Phillipa found herself in a triad between a weak husband and a manipulative and sadly underconfident daughter:

> 66 Amy continues to get from me the help she thinks she needs to sustain her life statement – which is 'I can't'. She can't drive, she can't find a job, she can't keep a boyfriend. But, you see, I feel that as a loving mother I *should* sympathize with her. In fact, Amy controls me expertly: she knows she can count on my feeling guilty if I say 'no' to her demands, so I cancel my own plans and ferry her about.
>
> As for my dependent husband, he uses a subtle form of pressure based on my being afraid that if I go off for a holiday with a girlfriend, he will collapse with some illness or other. He's done it several times, and each time I fall for it because I dare not risk really failing him as a dutiful wife. I should never forgive myself if he collapsed and died while I was away. Yes, they've both got me where they want me – at their beck and call. But they know I dare not tell them I've had enough. It's a pretty unhealthy, stagnant situation, isn't it?
>
> (personal communication) 99

Phillipa feels better now about herself (though she still sometimes guiltily contemplates rebellion) by refusing where she can to get hooked into her daughter's need for control. By being a kind, self-sacrificing wife and mother most of the time, she convinces herself she has done penance for the days she occasionally breaks out and refuses to go along with her family's requests. But her childhood conditioning is deeply entrenched. Therapy has loosened some of it, but in Phillipa's case going speedily to the core of the problem has not yielded speedy enough results.

CASE STUDY

An adopted child

Zak was the only child of an adoptee who showed her son no affection (presumably, receiving scant tenderness from her own adoptive parents). She and her husband had slept in separate rooms for as long as he could remember. When his father grew sick with Parkinson's Disease and was admitted to hospital, ten-year-old Zak was kept uninformed of his father's progress.

Then one month later his mother suddenly announced, 'Your father died last week.' Zak was not allowed to attend the funeral (not uncommon in the 1950s) and he had to wait until his fifties before he was able to mourn fully his father's death, learning in therapy to express his rage at his mother's irresponsible treatment. (The use of euphemism is another example of faulty thinking from the past. I have heard clients still grieving over a parent's death, remembering they were told by the surviving parent that the deceased had 'gone over the hill', or 'gone to a better place'. This obfuscation is not only bewildering for a child, waiting hopefully for more news, but damaging in its dishonesty.)

While he was growing up Zak suffered from nightmares, which started when his mother left him alone once weekly to play bingo and stop out late with friends. She gave him no explanation to account for her absence and he felt guilty that he should have felt so frightened when he first realized the house was empty. But his fear of being alone did not leave him until he went to university.

Later, in his twenties, he was attracted unerringly (as we have discussed in an earlier chapter) to a woman who was unconsciously playing out his projection of mother. Magnetized by the lure of the familiar, he too was ultimately to be shut out of his wife's bedroom. His lack of a more robust upbringing – with no strong male model – forced his compliance, just as his father had been forced to comply with his cold wife's demands for sexual abstinence.

Before he had finished therapy, Zak remarked, 'I see how all that pain in my family created the schizoid splits in them and in me. My late father feels much closer to me nowadays: he was a rejected man, just like I was for six years. My hope is that my two sons will alter the pattern, and form loving relationships with women only too willing to share their lives – and their bedrooms – with them, as they deserve.'

CASE STUDY

Playing it down

When the Robinsons (not their real name) began to realize they had parented a highly intelligent son, they quietly celebrated. Bruce was all they had dreamed of: charming, witty, ultra-bright and clearly destined for a stellar future. His little sister Emma, blue-eyed, biddable and pretty but showing no sign of her brother's ability, grew up to be sidelined by the brilliant boy. She recalls:

66 Rather than fail in holding my own against the shining sibling, I reasoned it was better not to try. My parents never said I was *not*

brainy, but in the light of no positive affirmation of any skill – artistic, linguistic, creative – on my part, I assumed I wasn't worthy to be encouraged like Bruce was encouraged, and with expensive hardware. I got cuddles but no affirmation. I got gifts too, but couldn't help noticing that Bruce was given presents worth thousands (computers, a piano) while I was given gerbils and roller blades, all things I wanted and had asked for at the time, yet never in the same league.

(personal communication) 99

In due course, after taking her GCSE examinations, Emma was astounded to open the results envelope and see four A*, four A and two B grades. Instantly, she thought, 'There's nothing wrong with me after all – there it is, on paper! And yet I still believed I was useless, because my parents didn't change their behaviour at home.' She went on:

66 When I achieved good A-level results and went on to university I was pathetically in need of people saying 'You have done well!' because I never got that sort of praise growing up. Bruce probably didn't either: but he was so obviously brilliant. Not that they ever said anything cruel, such as my brother was a genius and I was a thick idiot. It's just that in my childhood what were hurtful were the omissions, not what they said. Perhaps if I had been less sensitive, none of those subtle lacks would have mattered. But I think they blocked my route to real achievement, because by the time the penny had dropped that I wasn't a thick idiot, it was too late. I do recall, however, Mum saying my exam results rather surprised them. Not that she wasn't pleased for me, of course. Nowadays, I have to remind myself I have two degrees, that I must therefore be intelligent. Yet I can't own those achievements to anyone.

(personal communication) 99

Emma went on to marry and have children, determined to give both girls equal amounts of attention and admiration. The formula she believes she needed ('You are perfect as you are') she now offers to her two daughters, convinced this will forge their self-confidence throughout life. Her story is salutary, for no one involved in her history was at fault, certainly not in the quality of the overall loving care and involvement both Emma and Bruce received from their parents. Where faulty thinking seems to have crept in lies – as she has already offered from her perspective – in their keeping silent, failing to communicate the pride they felt in their daughter.

Perhaps Emma's parents themselves inherited a pattern of behaviour which left no room for lavish praise or verbal affirmation. As neither had been inculcated with such emotional literacy, they found it hard to summon up unfamiliar words in the domestic context, however deeply they felt about their gifted offspring. This is the legacy of the past.

A child psychiatrist (whose name I cannot now recall) once told me that his best results, working 50 years ago with his young patients, came from his slowly building up a relationship of trust with them. The key to it all, he urged (speaking as if for the distressed child) was: 'Call me good and praise me, and I *will* be good.' Half a century ahead of his time, he would surely have approved of Emma's twenty-first century belief system, with its power to nourish and encourage.

Summary

Behaviour, both good and bad, is passed down from generation to generation. Where there was poverty, lack of education, fear, or cultural, social tenets which held that children should barely be seen, let alone respected, we often see (by present-day standards) dysfunctional families. We are indeed the product of our conditioning, as the Indian philosopher Jiddu Krishnamurti stressed in *The Awakening of Intelligence* (1987), and during his talks worldwide during the last century. Slowly, people are learning to alter the patterning they inherited, opening up to the possibility of a more rewarding emotional outlook.

This is where counsellors and psychotherapists can work usefully, urging clients to retrace their histories to understand better how their behaviour has been influenced by their upbringing. When they begin to question the long-held views of their family ways, change can happen; but for reasons of imagined safety some, unfortunately, choose not to question them, preferring the security of the familiar.

Uncomfortable issues get pushed metaphorically under the carpet; difficult encounters get dodged; challenging matters are shrugged off with comments such as 'That's the way we do it.' Such rigidity can be frustrating for the practitioner, who may long to show their client how much more they might find in their lives by opening up to change. The use of encouraging phrases to nudge them on – such as 'Like . . .?', or 'It's as if . . .?' or 'For instance . . .?' and 'Suppose you *did* say/do such-and-such, what would happen next?' – can be helpful tools. It is often surprising how such phrases make clients focus on the kind of treatment or attitudes shown them in childhood to which they had so long inured themselves.

In the next chapter we explore the cost of collusion when couples stay together, finding themselves trapped in a loveless or hateful relationship, and for whom separation seems either impossible or less preferable of the two options.

7 Staying together expediently: the cost of collusion

Relationships do survive, despite the weight of submerged material, inherited damage and individual trauma. Statistics currently reflect a picture in which just over half the married population stay together; and we could presume the same applies to civil partnerships, although we have no evidence to confirm this. It is likely, therefore, that a large number of people in heterosexual and homosexual relationships continue their life together precisely because they like it that way or (as we will see later) sometimes because it is expedient to do so.

If we look at horses grazing in a field they demonstrate a basic need for closeness, a drive for creature comfort which humans also share. Originally, animals (and humans) grouped together for primal safety against attack, yet they obviously do so now for social reasons. We see horses grooming each other, nibbling inaccessible areas on the other's skin; swishing flies off heads with their tails; we hear them whinnying when one has has been taken out of the paddock, relaxing only when they are reunited. Such attachment behaviour parallels in effect the human state. If contented coexistence is not, however, the binding agent in a relationship, then we move into different psychological territory, where the animal kingdom has no place. Unlike people, animals have no taste for subtle forms of intrigue, for manipulation, or for self-deception. Their communication is clear: they show their feelings directly and act upon them unequivocally.

In the human arena, when a couple discover their relationship no longer holds the same charm it once did, they are less likely to declare their feelings immediately, or to act upon them without some painful reflection. They may find themselves faced with unpalatable decision making. Should they continue to put up with the situation, change it, or end the relationship? Not all couples come to the realization at the same time (if at all) that the marriage or partnership is no longer working. (Let us recall Betty in Chapter 2, the woman oblivious to her husband's sense of suffocation and her astonishment when he left her.) But usually, clues are there for both partners to witness and, perhaps, summon the courage to talk about them. Acknowledging the newly developing situation, however, can be daunting. Many, like Betty, will unconsciously deafen or blind themselves; or at least like countless others hope the problem will go away so that they will not have to deal with it. If it does not go away, then we move into the complex, shadowy land of collusion, as one partner or the other tries to hold on to the status quo.

Before going any further, it should be pointed out that to a lesser or greater extent we are all 'guilty' of acting collusively, or choosing the path of expediency, sometime in our lives. We might face reluctance to upset the home regime, family matters or career possibilities, and consciously opt for collusion or expediency. We shrug and accept, grin and bear it, put up with unpalatable situations until they can change. It is a matter of degree here. But when neurosis is woven subtly into these various situations we are likely to be blind to the real issues at stake, and this could be where danger lurks.

For those who unconsciously take the path of passivity, unaware of the cost involved to themselves as they ignore the stagnancy in their lives and their own true needs, their rationale will run on very different lines. Self-delusion will almost certainly lie behind that rationale; and we must not rule out ignorance, lack of insight, fearfulness. Sadly, this can nonetheless prove a far greater peril than they realize, for staying in an unhappy situation damages psychological health and quite possibly physical health.

Collusion is dishonest

In my copy of *Collins English Dictionary* (2009), the word 'collusion' is described as a secret agreement for a fraudulent purpose; connivance; conspiracy. That would be a definition to apply to the external world. But here, concerned as we are with inner world material, we must use the word collusion in its psychological sense, not readily found in dictionaries. Two people do not need to speak to one another implicitly to agree on a fraudulent purpose, there may be no joint acknowledgement, or whispered conspiracy together. Yet when one partner colludes with another they are both guilty of emotional dishonesty. Let us look at an example of collusion.

A couple has been married for ten years. They have two children and though not particularly enjoying their lives have found a way of existing as a family. The wife is the first to feel restless and decides to take up her job again as a laboratory assistant. There she meets and falls in love with a colleague, encouraging him to bring his wife home for regular dinners, and eventually all four adults go on annual holidays together.

Vaguely aware that he is being manipulated into colluding with these intimate meetings, the husband feels hurt and slightly suspicious, but naively goes along with the charade because by this time (a few years later) he too has taken a fancy to a work colleague. It suits him secretly to conduct his own affair, guessing his wife is similarly engaged, although she continues to protest her innocence. Nothing is said and there is no communication between them about the situation. As a schizoid personality type, he can largely split off from the rejection he feels, though aware that he had sought comfort elsewhere to assuage his grief at a disappointing marriage.

Eventually, inevitably, his wife's neat plan goes rotten. First to collapse under the strain of leading dissembling lives, the laboratory assistant lover falls seriously sick with cancer and dies. The callow husband by now has been made redundant at work, finds employment away from home and barely talks to his wife when he returns for weekends. Then he too feels unwell and puts that down to the shock of redundancy in mid-life. But he has developed a form of cancer, one in which long-term stress is said to play a major part.

Collusion played a big part also in this sorry tale, which is a true story. If the couple had found the emotional literacy to communicate their feelings in the early stages, risking rows instead of repressing difficult material, then a great deal of despair might have been avoided. The husband (now returned fully to health, leading a different life and in personal therapy) has since commented, 'I see how naive I was in failing to challenge my wife, and discuss the situation. I behaved like an adolescent – innocent, self-absorbed – wrongly thinking that as I was getting my own needs met on the side, silence was easier than confronting what was going on in my marriage.'

In *The Type C Connection: The Behavioral Links to Cancer and Your Health*, a book co-authored with Henry Dreher, American psychologist Lydia Temoshok asks the question in her introduction:

> 66 Can emotions and behavior affect our risk of cancer, or our recovery should we contract the disease? After a decade of study, I am convinced that a specific behavior pattern, which I have named 'Type C', does indeed alter both cancer risk and recovery. My own results converged with findings from scores of other published studies to paint a striking picture of how the mind may influence cancer development. . . . After talking with scores of patients for many hours over several months, I detected a striking and very specific behavior pattern among them. I arrived at the rather unnerving realization that almost all the patients were extremely nice.
> (1992: 3–4) 99

Temoshok found they were unwilling to disappoint; devoted to pleasing their spouses, parents, siblings, friends or co-workers. Their very identity seemed to depend wholly upon the reflected acceptance of those people significant in their lives, 'other-directed' and in denial, with an under-developed sense of self ('I'm fine – it's my wife/husband I'm worried about'); out of touch with their primary needs and emotions, they look to others for signals on how to think, feel and act.

Unhealthy foursome

The husband discussed above, who colluded with his wife's manipulative plans to see more of her lover, clearly falls into this group; as did the other husband involved, a man whose unloved wife was an alcoholic but from whom he was unwilling to part (another collusive act) because he liked the security of domestic routine, despite the drinking episodes. Of course, this example of collusion on both men's parts for the duration of the unhealthy foursome does not always mean a formula for disaster. Other couples have managed to survive collusive situations or arrangements and come out in some cases stronger and wiser (more of this later). But to return to Temoshok:

> 66 Many factors govern the readiness, sensitivity, and vigor of our immune defences. Our genes are the first and foremost influence on immunity. Environmental agents affect immunity, and so do our dietary habits. Now research in the young field of psychoneuro-immunology teaches us that our behavior patterns and mind states also affect the immune system. We finally have scientific proof that the mind plays a part in the activity of our vital natural defences. . . . In brief, the linkage involves brain chemicals called *neurotransmitters* and *neuropeptides*. They are literally the chemical carriers of emotion. Neurotransmitters are discharged by nerve cells, and when an emotion is aroused in us, they act on other cells throughout the brain and body, causing all sorts of physiologic changes.
>
> (1992: 67–8) 99

A strong point here to support the husband's own insightful retrospection comes with Temoshok's research into why men and women with Type C patterns often get sick. She insists that patients are seldom aware of their Type C behaviour; that if aware they may not recognize it as a psychological impediment, or that it could affect their health. She suggests they do not realize they can change their behaviour, which is unconscious and unintentional. Going into psychotherapy, they slowly understand their injurious patterning. She adds:

> 66 Once embarked on a process of change, most Type C patients forgive themselves for past mistakes, patterns, feelings, or relationships over which they feel shame. They recognize how deeply ingrained was their pattern, how ignorant they

were of its ill effects, and how difficult it is to change. They develop, to borrow Lawrence LeShan's phrase, 'a fierce and tender concern for every part of themselves', especially for the child within who stifled needs and feelings in order to maintain harmony in his home.

(1992: 233–4) **99**

This is a perceptive observation and one which, although here pertaining to health, is central to the theme of *Relationship Therapy*, where early distortions and suppressed feelings are seen as bedrock to psychological breakdown in adulthood. Because the two couples in my case study were all damaged by their upbringing, they found themselves unable – or unwilling – to address current problems, preferring to go with expediency and with familiar covert ways of being. The strain involved over several years undoubtedly caused ill health; a terrible cost and (although genetic predisposition must top the determining factors list) one, possibly, which could have been avoided.

Relate's Barbara Bloomfield offers another view of health issues occurring in some dysfunctional relationships. She reports:

66 There are some couples who manage staying together very well: for example, one becomes the carer for the other, the situation suiting them. We often see psychosomatic illness coming up. Systemically, the illness serves a function by acting as a homeostatic mechanism, to keep things going the way they are. A wife might say 'I know I am a misery guts, but I do have this heart murmur (or whatever)', and that's the way her depression, or temper, becomes bearable, so serving them both.

(personal communication) **99**

CASE STUDY
Without options

Lara, a Seattle mother of three, was married to a successful American businessman who provided his family with a large house with six bedrooms, private country club membership and a rich lifestyle many would envy. Indeed, women friends probably envied Lara in the way Jim came home every evening without fail, wanting his little girls (all under four years old) tucked up in bed so that he could enjoy the evening entirely alone with his wife.

Jim frowned on incoming or outgoing telephone calls to the house after teatime. If Lara was answering a call and heard the garage doors opening, she would immediately hang up because Jim had explained it took time away from him: she could understand that, and at first felt treasured. But the possessiveness got worse. He wanted no sign of his daughters once he was back from work. He would get angry to see toys anywhere, or find even a hairband on the floor; once he threatened if that happened again, he would cut off the child's hair. It did, and he did.

Jim's need for control insidiously attacked Lara's ability to see through it. So she colluded with his demands in order to keep the peace. By now the demands were excessive, with Jim insisting no household chores should be done after five o'clock. All he wanted was to sit watching television with his wife. If she had parked the family car in the garage with the wheels turning to the right, it would be wrong; if to the left, the same. The front door key should hang on this hook, not that one – how could she be so haphazard, unreliable? Lara describes what she calls her warped sense of reality at this point, how she feared she was losing her mind:

> By now, I was beginning to realize too he was making the girls feel no respect for me – how could they, when all they heard from their father was if I 'just behaved' he wouldn't have to get so mad at me. Or, if I weren't so stupid, he wouldn't continually have to correct me. I began to think he must be right. Then one evening, we went out to eat at a restaurant. Jim complained endlessly about the drinks, the meal, and in the end the manager gave us a complimentary bill and asked that we never come back there.
>
> I often heard strangers comment 'How can she stand it?' and still I hadn't the courage to leave him. I just didn't realize I had that option. We moved house every two years so I was isolated from my own family and unable to sustain friendships, just when I needed them most. On my fortieth birthday, with the kids in the car, Jim wouldn't let me climb in. I kept trying and he'd drive on a bit. I began to cry, still holding on to the car, then he'd go on a little bit further while the kids were themselves crying. Jim thought the whole thing was a great laugh.
>
> (personal communication)

Often feeling suicidal, Lara eventually packed a suitcase for herself and the girls and went to stay with an old friend. It had taken her a year to plan her escape (as she puts it) but she omitted telling the children because she was afraid if Jim learned of her plan he would himself commit suicide. When Lara started seeing a psychotherapist, admitting her fears for Jim, the therapist retorted, 'Jim is homicidal, not suicidal. You had better be very, very careful.'

The divorce court gave her full custody with no visitation, the girls not seeing their father again for a number of years. She and the children went through intensive therapy during the intervening time and developed skill sets Lara wished she had possessed herself when trying to deal with Jim during the marriage. As Lara says, 'He doesn't treat them now as he once treated me. They simply wouldn't allow it. That is what was so difficult, realizing I should have been able to avoid this if I had been smarter, or braver.'

After two years in psychotherapy, Lara felt she had achieved little ('I was too tired, too afraid'), aware she was still scared of Jim and disgusted with herself for her collusive cowardice. But then one day she suddenly raged violently in session as she and her therapist discussed her middle daughter recently bullying her ('My therapist, Hank, was of course thrilled!'), and she had found the breakthrough needed. She discovered the value of therapy and insisted she stay on, although her elderly practitioner was on the point of retirement, postponing this (as he later admitted) because he wanted professionally to see her complete her work.

CASE STUDY

Material dependence

When Cordelia met Simon at a drinks party she was drawn to this tall, powerful man with a strong sexual magnetism. Both were married to other people, yet both found the lacks in their existing relationships sufficiently strong that they decided, in time, to leave their spouses. Simon had been regularly cuckolded by his *puella* wife, bent on taking lovers in the same way she might go shopping for new clothes. Cordelia, on the other hand, after a long marriage to a man much older than herself, was no longer finding her needs as a woman were being met. It was almost inevitable that she and Simon would find consolation together.

They set up home in Cordelia's elegant house, bought from her elderly husband, Alistair, and contracted in Simon's name. In those days, there was a great deal of money around; Simon was a rich man and Cordelia's husband felt reassured she would have a comfortable life. There was no financial settlement, therefore. Then Alistair remarried.

For the next few years, waiting for Simon's own divorce to come through, the lovers faced many crises, exacerbated by the fact of Simon's schizoid character structure. Whenever he felt himself under any kind of perceived attack, he withdrew behind his emotional carapace. Cordelia (echoing the theme of the schizoid/hysteric partnership described in Chapter 4) became frantic in her attempts to bring him out of that split-off place. The more she begged him to remember she was neither his controlling ex-wife nor his insensitive, unloving mother, the more he 'disappeared'. His adult children were often painfully rude to her, yet he failed to support Cordelia on such occasions.

> 66 When this happened, my sense was he was so frightened of losing his children's love if he tried to defend me, he couldn't really value himself properly to tell them they should care about his happiness and stop being rude to me. He longed for their approval and was very wary about making our relationship permanent by marrying me, knowing how much they hated the idea. I began to feel deeply insecure about my position. Finally, however, we did get married. For two or three years we were actually all right together, although he was away a great deal on business. Then there was trouble with his company: in an effort to put it back on track, Simon mortgaged our house – MY house since I was first married to Alistair – insisting it was the only solution. I was very, very angry.
>
> (personal communication) 99

Simon took to his carapace again, barely acknowledging Cordelia's distress at the real possibility she would lose her old home if his company did collapse. Materially dependent on him, she realized she had nothing after walking away from Alistair 22 years earlier without a settlement or a career and now would have little money to live on if she left Simon. 'It was an appalling situation I'd got myself into, but I said to myself I'd made my bed and I was going to lie in it. And I still had hope Simon would turn to me emotionally again.'

Staying with him was an expedience. Here was a 60-year-old woman, facing old age with a man who was increasingly demonstrating his unconscious dislike and distrust of women. The two he had once trusted had betrayed him (mother and former wife) and here was the third, his present wife, on whom he began to project his childhood rage and spite, surfacing at last as his business stresses brought out his own deep insecurities. As we have seen before, it often takes a crisis to prompt long-buried trauma to emerge from the unconscious. Cordelia was in the firing line.

A year later she asked for a divorce, putting an end to her uneasy life with Simon. All hope gone, she managed to come out of her miserable existence with enough capital to purchase a small house and live modestly, far removed from the decades of affluence she had known. Today, Cordelia is wiser and stronger for her bitter experience. Therapy has helped her come to terms with her grief ('I mourn as much for Simon as for myself: he has had so little joy in his life, even if he was skilled at splitting off to avoid pain') and she is on course for more emotionally rewarding relationships in the future. As psychotherapist Wyn Bramley says in *Bewitched, Bothered and Bewildered*:

> 66 Revisiting the past cannot change that past, but its losses and sadnesses can be faced, mourned, and laid to rest. As a result, future relationships are no longer compromised, burdened by old ghosts. They stand a much better chance of surviving; not only because less impossible expectation is placed upon them, but also because the very choice of partner will have been beneficially affected by having dealt with past trauma.
>
> (2008: 214) 99

This was certainly true of Cordelia, who could view her long affair-cum-marriage with Simon with realism at last. She resolutely moved on to forge other relationships and has since found happiness, no longer burdened by old ghosts. Achieving that new state, however, was not easy.

As Cordelia looked back over her frustrating life with Simon she realized how much it had damaged her self-esteem. 'He was offered a lovely way of life with me, and he chose not to take it. I sometimes felt I was an inconvenience; that he was torn between his need to be with me, and pleasing his adult children. They were the only constant in his life – as he perceived it – and perhaps the only people he believed he could trust. His selling our home, trying to salvage the business, was tied up with wanting to please them. It was all very sad.'

As Bramley states:

> 66 Melancholia in mid-life is extremely common, and is almost always bound up with frustrated hopes and a sense of wasted time and opportunity. We all need to make sense of our lives, find meaning in it, if we are to stay psychologically well. You can love someone all your adult life and not fully know them until they start getting restless or withdrawn in mid-life, and in the mid-life of your marriage to them. They are unable to tell you what is wrong because very often *they do not know themselves*.
>
> (2008: 136) 99

CASE STUDY
When collusion works

Barry and his partner Eva prided themselves on having the best of all worlds. In return for his devotion to their marriage, Barry was permitted the occasional public flirtation with any pretty woman who chose to play the same game with him. There were times when Eva did feel jealous (her husband was attractively seductive), but forced herself to leave the party on her own or retire to bed earlier than he wanted to, still absorbed elsewhere. She earned his praise next day, always laughing off his flirtatious ways as 'Barry's harmless fun'. Presenting a mature facade, not that far removed from being indulgent Good Mother, suited her idea of a good marriage. It also, of course, suited Barry.

Eva looked upon his behaviour with other men's wives or girlfriends as innocuous. She guessed it was some kind of ongoing test of his pulling power in the male competitive arena, but she believed him when he said he never took the flirtations to the next level. He loved her, and constantly told her so, always pleased when she managed to look good without make-up, hair-styling or smart clothes. Flattered that he saw her as the woman above all others with whom he chose to live, it never occurred to her that his behaviour was self-centred; that applauding her for looking dowdy actually ensured there might be less chance of her finding admirers too. He wanted the game played strictly to his rules.

This charade went on over the years, never destabilizing the marriage. It seemed the collusion worked and even if there were strands of self-deception in the mix. After all, no harm had been done; they were still happy together. Then, a decade or so later, an ex-neighbour's student daughter came to stay with them on her way to look over a new university. Barry enjoyed her company and, on hugging her farewell, could not resist placing a hand over her breast and giving it a few squeezes. The visitor said nothing, all farewells completed. Within a week, however, Barry and Eva received an outraged letter. In therapy, Eva said, 'We were amazed! I mean, Barry didn't mean any harm, it was just a bit of fun. Why anyone should take exception to such a little thing beats me – it was obviously only a friendly joke.'

I reflected back that this young woman did not seem to be taking his behaviour as a joke, that she sounded angry and upset. She had also said she viewed this as an assault, which was a criminal offence. She had pointed out he had not only abused her, but also his role as host and trusted former neighbour. What were Eva's feelings now about her husband's part in this? She unhesitatingly replied, 'I'm cross with the girl, actually – fancy telling him off for just touching her in a friendly, jokey way. I didn't think it was bad when I saw him do it, I wasn't worried a bit.'

A lifetime's collusion with a self-indulgent husband had reduced Eva's personal integrity to shreds. So laden with self-delusion was she that she failed to see the enormity of what had happened to their visitor and their earlier long-term relationship. Eva had now become wrapped up in denial. As Walker says in *Surviving Secrets*:

> 66 Denial and resistance are powerful aspects of the psychology both of the individual and, collectively, of society. Both defences come strongly into play if the beliefs and values of either are threatened. Abuse can be, and in effect is, denied, both by those who perpetrate it and by others. The ability of abusers to deny their behaviour, even when presented with incontrovertible evidence, is astounding.
>
> (1992: 2) 99

So collusion did not destroy Eva and Barry. As Bloomfield sees it: 'Some couples stay together because although they may not have very happy patterns, they have made their relationship work.' She adds:

> 66 After all, what is a totally wonderful relationship? Has anyone of us really had it? Intimacy, love, sex, being allowed to feel safe to be yourself, to be able to go away from base to do things with other people without jealousy (such as separation for business, or different holiday destinations) – surely we might say that that is good enough?
>
> (personal communication) 99

Summary

Facing pitfalls when they occur in relationships can be, as we have seen time and again, painful and difficult. Those who find the courage to meet and do battle with them are the clients who emerge all the stronger for the experience; they have learned how and why much of their distress was caused. Some will ultimately choose new lives; others will prefer to try to hold on to the status quo, no matter the cost to their personal integrity. It is not the therapist's job to enforce change – more, to facilitate new ways of thinking wherever possible.

Though seldom discussed in psychology's literature, collusion is a corrosive element in any relationship. It can work seemingly well in keeping a marriage together, but the partnership will be based on fraudulent values and these could carry an implicit threat to mental health. What works for one may do immense harm to the other. Often it is only when the victim of a collusive or expedient partnership presents themselves for therapy that the web of psychological deceit can begin to be untangled; and then not always successfully.

How does the counsellor or therapist address the problem of collusion? First, there is the need to identify it ensnared in a couple. Glaringly obvious in

Eva's case, where she shifted her focus on to blaming the innocent young student, we see that her paramount wish is to keep viewing her husband in a good light. In doing so, she ensures her own position of emotional security, loved by a man she sees as admirable. Thinking as one, they are therefore unassailable.

The therapist's task is to keep questioning her reasoning, perhaps gently to challenge the rigidity, offer other ways of looking at a situation. At some level, Eva will know there is cause for concern. Co-dependency (as in their marriage) provides fertile psychological soil for self-delusion, each partner backing up the other to serve their own needs. I have found that exploring how as children they related to their carers (was having to please them involved?) can help start a process of separating out crucial dependency issues.

Only when a client is ready to think for themselves, to question their own real needs, are they able to examine what they truly want out of life. Unconsciously, they may feel anger at being coerced into collusion (or expedient practice), controlled by others; they submit because they see, as in childhood, no other way.

The risk of head-on confrontation is too great for many people to contemplate, and so they collude with the bullying tactics in their partner, however neatly disguised. Using Gestalt methods (the empty chair, or chairs) to speak to an imaginary parent or partner can prove effective; or acting out being those characters, hopefully to ignite the embers of rage so well repressed in the psyche. This can sometimes be triggered by inviting the client to imagine a typical scenario, asking what would happen next if they had showed their hurt or rebelliousness. Then work with the new material surfacing.

Cognitive understanding holds a valuable place in such work. If a practitioner can, at some appropriate point, explain the overview as she or he sees it, there is a good chance a client will also see the truth of that overview. For example: 'I'm wondering if you might not feel Barry needs you, somehow, to believe his every word? He's less likely to be abandoned by you if he keeps assuring you of his love, praising you for exceptional intelligence grasping his deep philosophies (which, by the way, include rubbishing the need for necessary new clothes and lipstick). Does this really feel right to you? No? So is there anything you'd like to say to him at this moment, if he were in the room?'

Ill health can result from an unhappy partner staying in an abusive, manipulative or futile relationship. This is a sensitive issue, but important for the therapist to remember, should later sessions continue to confirm an unhealthy stasis. Steering the client to consult their GP might be indicated here, particularly if the client expresses concern over any symptoms.

In the next and final chapter, we discover some long-standing relationships which worked and continue to flourish, and where communication and self-awareness have eased them through the painful patches.

8 When relationships work successfully

There was an old newsroom saying in my cub reporting days that couples interviewed on the occasion of their golden wedding anniversary would invariably offer as their recipe for staying happily married together for 50 years: 'Give and take!' Now it seems they were right. That simple attitude actually does lie behind the most successful relationships, a union where some sort of balance has been achieved and maintained. But what those elderly country folk did not reveal during their encounter with the press was the emotional pain, the sheer hard work that it had probably taken for them to reach their enviable position of contentment.

When it came to choosing whom to ask for these final case study interviews, I found an extraordinarily rich seam of material emerging from – it must be said – the most unexpected sources. People who had made their relationships work only after a great deal of effort; men and women who wondered how they could endure another day or week locked in the distress their partnership was causing them; two men who reached breaking point before they found a solution to their seemingly insuperable problem of jealousy; a travel writer who realized one step further in the rows she and her husband were having would mean catastrophic changes neither wanted.

The theme common to all these stories was that peace was hard won, that the value of giving and taking from each other proved the binding force, and that a state of harmony was the prize that lay at the end of their commitment. Hardly surprising perhaps, when we reflect on the content of earlier chapters, where subpersonalities, inherited faulty thinking, damaged childhood, trauma, neuroses and so on all played a part in forging attitudes to adult experience.

Yet despite all this, more couples stay together than break up. Relationships are complex, their success or failure based on multifactorial issues, where they can work for indefinable reasons or fail for comparatively trivial reasons. This book has been written to try to point out the more likely causes for breakdown and to offer guidelines for practitioners. It cannot explain, however, why some couples solve their own problems, do not ask for – or need – professional help, and succeed spectacularly when even the private lives of counsellors and therapists may teeter and fall.

Spirit of our times

So we have a couples situation where there are some surprises, some disappointments, but also a constancy which continues to reflect the wishes of the majority. Yet we cannot deny that the twenty-first century may increasingly demonstrate a different pattern. Young and old are exposed to ever more choice and temptation, where change is considered acceptable in ways once deemed inappropriate. Men and women say to themselves nowadays 'This isn't working' and move on (without much reflection) to new situations. Complex living arrangements abound. Bloomfield points out the inherent dangers lying in this prevailing mindset:

> At Relate, without being prescriptive saying what a relationship should be, we say to clients just look at what you have got, before you take another step. People jump into new things, it's the zeitgeist, the spirit of our times. I see children who tell me their complicated lives, they don't know who they are any longer. A young person will tell me 'Last year I had my own bedroom, a dog, but now I am living in a different house, sharing a bedroom with a new stepsister, my dog was given away because the stepsister's got allergies, and I never see my father/mother.' If we think about attachment needs, perhaps we should consider how amazing it is that people attach so well, considering how complex their home arrangements are.
>
> (personal communication)

Bloomfield has been with her partner Ben for 30 years. They enjoyed the good times and got through the bad times. Their relationship continues to hold potential, as she says, because they are intellectually well matched, interested in the same cultural pursuits. When they have rows, they have learned not to say to each other 'Oh, God! I've heard that before,' but instead say something along the lines of 'What you're saying is important, but I'm not getting it, even though I'm sure there's something in what you are saying.'

She adds: 'That sense of possibility, of yearning, is still with us, which keeps us going, whereas a lot of people just finish because they are so fed up they don't want to be in the same house, or even country. In that case, at Relate we might urge a week apart, suggest they go and visit a friend. The need then is to pull apart, not part company.'

When psychotherapist Richard Hycner sees a warring couple for the first time, he speaks of three faults which tend to lie behind their unhappiness: disconnection, disappointment and disillusionment. He calls that The Blame Game, an impasse which a therapist must de-escalate. He points out to his clients that underneath the blame a partner is unconsciously making a statement: 'You are not connected to me as I want you to be.' Blaming is part of the negative cycle which interrupts dialoguing. Talking to therapists at a seminar in England in 2009 he added:

> 66 Ask yourself what's behind that blame? What's behind each partner's hurt and injury – this is the role of repairing the function. Ask yourself what is the pattern which is keeping these people stuck? Don't see an individual first and then as part of a couple: I tell each person there is no confidentiality, because I make available information in the room between the three of us. Attunement is vital to both people, so that one or the other isn't frightened off. Deal with this gingerly, for part of the artistry of therapy is to ask yourself if you are focussing too much on Mary, how is John dealing with this? There is a danger in isolating the other person. Allow your gut reaction, your sense about what's going on, to guide the session.
>
> (personal communication) 99

Hycner went on to suggest that there can be no intimacy in a relationship without vulnerability, that clients have to trust themselves to take small risks, then they can be more willing to take the next risk to build something creative. 'The paradox in a situation where one partner is desperate to get the other to change is in learning that the only person we can change is ourself, and in so doing it actually produces change in the other.'

CASE STUDY
A triad relationship

Justin, now in his late sixties, could be said to fit somewhere into this generalized description observed by Hycner. Over a period of many years, loving Miranda in a triad relationship with Owen, and unable to claim her undivided attention, Justin realized his only hope of peace was to change his own view of what seemed a hopeless situation. He found himself in an 'on/off' regimen, where he could revel in the joy of being with her exclusively, only to learn that her other lover, Owen, would be arriving later in the day. Painfully, he withdrew, unable to make Miranda see clearly that the triad would not, could not give her lasting happiness. She takes up their story:

> 66 I had got caught in Owen's web. As a single parent with two boys to raise, I was only too glad to have Owen move into my life. He was fantastic with my sons, magical for me and in time I desperately wanted Owen to make a commitment to me permanently. He prevaricated, with 'yes/no' responses and then I saw there wasn't going to be a future with him. But nonetheless I felt trapped in a web: I was addicted to Owen. In the meantime, I met Justin. I enjoyed sex with him every bit as much as with Owen, yet still I just didn't seem able to get over my addiction.
>
> (personal communication) 99

Justin stayed away, miserable, and yet continued contact with Miranda, who wrote him dozens of distraught letters over the next few years. He tried relationships with other women, but his unhappiness would not go away. Meanwhile, Miranda took herself into psychotherapy. She reports:

> 66 What came out in the therapy was that I could not trust anyone, and set up constantly to be betrayed! It might have been father stuff [clinging on to Owen], but I never really did discover what lay behind my lack of trust. Perhaps the fact that I was seduced at 14 by someone living in my house (which I actually welcomed and continued that relationship for the next 15 years) had something to do with the situation I put myself in with Owen. He seduced me, so a pattern was repeating itself. But behind it all was, I think, the fact that I needed two men to want me sexually: my self-worth was confirmed. To be desired by them both, for a long time, was a boost to my morale.
>
> (personal communication) 99

Helped by her therapist to understand that her relationship with Owen was (and always would be) hopeless, Miranda withdrew from both men. She moved house and went to live up country in order to send both her sons to the same school Justin's daughter had valued. The couple met once more, virtually as neighbours, living in cottages in the same village.

No longer feeling the need for excitement in a triad relationship, Miranda settled quietly into country life and was glad to renew contact with Justin who, in discarding his desperation over so many years to change her, had contributed to her psychological shift. Therapy had done the rest. All three members of the trio had worked with therapists individually on their awareness and understanding, and then as a working threesome to reflect upon their respective patterns of behaviour. Miranda concludes the story:

66 Justin and I got married over a decade ago, because we wanted to celebrate the fact that we were together, that the feelings were mutual. We had a lovely wedding at home, surrounded by our children, their partners, our grandchildren and our friends. I am being very nurtured now by Justin, able at last to receive the love he tells me he's felt for me for nearly 20 years. It won't be that long before I am in my seventies! I look back on that energetic dashing about all those years ago and remember mostly, I think, the sexual energy which drove Owen, Justin and me to do such crazy things. Sexual energy creates the motivation, but actually it's more complex than just sex: it was what lay underneath (my lack of trust) which kept me locked into having relationships with two men at the same time. There was a lot of love about: maybe it also fuelled an intense quality into our everyday life.

(personal communication) 99

CASE STUDY
Their own solution

Surrendering to the process of self-exploration and reflection formed a backdrop to open the way for Miranda and Justin to lead ultimately fuller lives, even if it took them to late mid-life to achieve emotional maturity and contentment together. But for another couple, Eddie and Arthur, the struggle to find peace meant finding a solution which at first sight appears to contradict the tenets discussed above. This couple feel now at their most comfortable and safe in their civil partnership by ensuring a third party joins them occasionally. Let Arthur explain:

66 It's stressful being gay: well, it was where I was born in Scotland. It was no easy ride for me to come to terms with it 20 years ago, and I said to myself as I looked around the gay bars in Scotland then, 'If this is how my life is going to pan out for the next half century, trying to find a relationship, I would rather be dead.' But I came south, met Eddie and we fell in love. Our respective university degrees and training made us complementary working partners as well as being lovers. So we began our own

> agency business, running it side by side very successfully. Before this, each of us travelling abroad and being parted a lot, we had grown distrustful of each other. Now, working and living together, we know what the other is up to.
>
> (personal communication) 99

The temptations in the homosexual world, the casual gay scene where youth and beauty are key criteria for quick sexual conquests meant for Arthur and Eddie countless painful quarrels. The years brought increasing opportunity for affairs, but both men realized that the subsequent showdowns when one or the other got found out made the excursions hardly worth the passing pleasure. Did they want an open relationship, like so many other gay couples? 'No, we did not. But we agreed it was abhorrent to imagine a lifetime of monogamy – yet what was the alternative, if we were to avoid the grief of rows and jealousy? Then Eddie said if we wanted other people involved, it must be for fun alone. Together, or not at all.'

So began a new era for the couple. Living in a lively gay community, they go out to city bars and occasionally meet a man they both like enough to invite him home. They tell him bluntly: 'This is strictly for fun, you are coming into our relationship and you must play it to our rules. If you don't like it, there's the door.' Arthur and Eddie believe they love each other deeply. They have been in the same relationship for 15 years and cannot imagine not living together for the rest of their lives. 'Why would we think of going off and having an affair when we have so much?' is their rationale. The solution they have found to resolve their agonies of insecurity when under threat from covert liaisons is working well for them. They have a secret code (two taps on the shoulder) to inform the other that a possible rendezvous with a newcomer is not acceptable; or if there is a hint that the sexual encounter might lead to future emotional entanglement they have a strict rule. Arthur said:

> 66 If we can see this could blow our relationship apart, then I put an ultimatum down and say 'You have to make a choice, him or me.' It's taken years to get to the point of believing we do have a good relationship and where we realize the implications of what it would mean if we split up. We know each other inside out, we like each other. Intimacy is precious to us both. There's been a psychological shift: our life now really *is* about give and take. The value of our relationship means we don't want anything to interfere, in any shape or form, which would take away what we have earned so painfully. If it did, it would have to be something monumental.
>
> (personal communication) 99

The couple both sought counselling during the difficult years of jealous quarrels. They went separately, each agreeing that talking through their respective distress with professionals helped them understand how they could arrive at a workable solution for themselves in learning to communicate their needs to each other and find acceptable strategies. As Arthur reflected, 'I came from a family in which my mother literally wouldn't speak to my father for days, months; they lived at opposite ends of the house. So I can hold a grudge much longer than Eddie can – I've been conditioned to it! But he goads me into discussing it, which is a good thing.'

How does this gay couple see their distant future together? 'We talk about pooling our resources with other gay friends, buying a mansion with lots of apartments and getting boys in to do the cooking and cleaning. Yes, we probably will end up living with friends who are also still together. We hope our nephews and nieces will want to come and visit, because there won't be any children to look after us when we're old,' Eddie said.

CASE STUDY

House husband

When freelance travel writer Cassie used to pack her bag and wave goodbye to the children at the window, neighbours in her street were worried. Her departures were noted; as were her returns, to loving hugs on the doorstep with her husband Ivan. But how many more times, the neighbours wondered, could the couple continue splitting up after what must have been a quarrel, then make up again, only to repeat the entire cycle a few months later? Nobody had told them about Cassie's job, since they seldom had conversations in the street. Yet the curtain twitching went on until one day another neighbour explained all. 'They're not constantly breaking up!' she exclaimed 'Ivan and Cassie are devoted to each other. But he stays at home, looking after the little ones, and she works for travel magazines and newspapers, so she's away at different times to write about faraway places.'

Cassie told me this in session, discussing perceptions and how mistaken people can be. Now in her seventies, retired from freelancing, her life is filled with helping look after several grandchildren living a hundred miles away. If she leaves home with a packed bag it is to give her daughter some respite: the children's father is in the armed forces and serving overseas. These days, Ivan still greets her with joyful hugs on her return; but nobody could guess how hard this welcome was won. No one knew the pain and disappointment they had experienced over the previous 20 years. It would be their secret from family and friends; for neither believed in talking about their struggles, least of all to a therapist: that would have been self-indulgent. 'We can work this out for ourselves!' was their robust motto. And work it out they did.

As Cassie explained:

> 66 We had rough times and big rows. Ivan got bored looking after the children, while I gallivanted (as he saw it) all over the world for editors. He gave up his own career to further mine, a house husband before it became the norm, which is probably why our neighbours could only see one scenario as they watched me leave home so many times. People in those days expected the man to go out to work, the woman to stay in with the children and bake cakes. Ivan and I were perfectly happy in principle about swapping roles, but although we made rational decisions about our lives, making sure our two girls were content with the routine, I realize neither of us thought through the psychological dangers behind our planning. As the years went by, Ivan became increasingly morose about his loss of status in the world.
>
> (personal communication) 99

Jealousy was not an issue. They discussed their feelings about infidelity and agreed that neither was prepared to risk their own relationship for the sake of a sexual involvement elsewhere. For them, Ivan's lack of fulfilment became the canker: he had no other outlet for his own abilities, rather no outlet that would not take him away from home and the consistent parenting their daughters needed throughout their school life. But frustration became the core issue of their increasing unhappiness together. Ivan could see no way forward without upsetting the family too drastically and reneging on his part of the domestic agreement. Cassie reflected:

> 66 We realized that one step further in our rows would lead us in the wrong direction and catastrophic changes. We absolutely did not want those changes. So we worked at our relationship, communicating, listening to each other, loving, generous in our understanding of the other's pain. Finally, sticking at it for as long as it took, we found peace. Now, we are content. We must have reached that state of *agape*, which the ancient Greeks described as following on to the time of eros, erotic love, in a couple's life.
>
> (personal communication) 99

So why did Cassie come into therapy, when she and her husband had achieved so much on their own? Might the reason have something to do with resolution, of confirming with an outsider the validity of their hard work? Cassie had, in first making contact to ask for an appointment, suggested our time together would probably only be brief, a few sessions at most. Recognizing this as a familiar remark some prospective clients make (often through anxiety or resistance), I quietly checked out if in due course there would be space for her should she later realize she wanted longer term therapy. There was no need to worry. Cassie had fewer than six sessions. Confirmation was what she wanted, and confirmation was what she got. She left wreathed in smiles, her manner light and confident.

Here was someone who, married to a man committed to talking difficulties through, had been both fortunate in finding her match and courageous too. As the emotional shocks, the disappointments and frustrations hit them both over nearly 50 years together, Cassie and Ivan had seamlessly moved to stand, as it were, on the spot marked by previous generations of golden wedding couples. Like the silver-haired men and women last century interviewed for their local newspaper, they too gave and took throughout their long relationship, silent to the outside world about their difficulties.

Would psychotherapy or couple counselling decades ago have made their lives any easier? The answer is probably 'yes', because as we have seen throughout insight into the world of the unconscious is important. But it is an equivocal 'yes'. Ivan may well have colluded with Cassie, preferring the safety of house husbanding to taking a risk, facing challenging professional hurdles of his own outside. Such collusion could eventually have fed into his morose feelings of low self-worth; depression being the likely outcome, suppressing his anger both at his wife and at himself. But they had come through their painful difficulties, as Cassie's brief time in therapy testified, confirming their self-sufficiency. I am minded here of that old saying 'If it ain't broke, don't fix it.' Their relationship had never actually broken down; they had hauled themselves back each time for the greater good. Maybe there are times when therapeutic intervention is not, after all, automatically indicated.

The will to succeed

There are many roads leading to psychological maturity or, as Jungian analysts would describe it, individuation. We have seen how some people achieve this with professional help, and how others appear to have achieved something resembling it without therapy. Contentment in a relationship rests largely upon the couple's level of commitment, a quality more rare in the twenty-first century but by no means dead, as Relate's Barbara Bloomfield reports. Relate counsellors hear two-thirds of their clients claim they want to remain in their existing relationship. Bloomfield again:

 In thousands of cases, I am often surprised how people do stay together. But their object relations arrangements are so entrenched, they are the ones who are the most likely to do so, even when the signs are that they are very unhappy.

I ask them 'How many years do you want to remain so unhappy? Can you bear to carry on like this – what about YOU here?' A lot of us compromise in our life, and some people make their relationship work precisely because they have made collusion work. Some, too, will consciously reject their own upbringing and do the reverse when it comes to raising their own children, and living amicably with their partner. So, despite all the changes and choices in the twenty-first century, I feel very positive about the future.

(personal communication) **99**

In conclusion

We have come a long way since the earlier discussions on the realms of the unconscious, our hidden controllers, subpersonalities, allies, demons and neuroses, and it is my hope that readers will understand better at this point just how much they all influence the quality of relationships, our ability to cope with them, or not; and the rich insights to be found if we choose to look beneath the surface.

We end with an apocryphal tale in which a Buddhist monk solemnly addresses a young couple preparing to get married. 'Marriage,' he says 'is about three rings. There is the engagement ring, the wedding ring, and there is the suffering.' In these modern times, when partners do not necessarily have use for gold or platinum bands, we do know, however, that suffering is likely to be an integral part of the deal. It is the human condition. Yet without suffering we would probably have no understanding, no opportunity for growth and development, no triumph over poor odds, no hope for change. We would, indeed, have no relationships of any real substance.

Now, that *would* be sad.

References

Attwood, T. (1998) *Asperger's Syndrome: A Guide for Parents and Professionals*. London: Jessica Kingsley Publishers.

Baker, R. (1995) *Understanding Panic Attacks and Overcoming Fear*. Oxford: Lion Publishing.

Bloomfield, B. (2009) *The Relate Guide to Finding Love*. London: Vermilion.

Bowlby, J. (1969–1975) *Attachment and Loss*. London: Hogarth Press.

Bramley, W. (2008) *Bewitched, Bothered and Bewildered*. London: Karnac Books.

Brown, D. and Pedder, J. (1979) *Introduction to Psychotherapy*. London: Tavistock Publications.

Casement, P. (1985) *On Learning from the Patient*. New York: Tavistock Publications.

Edwards, D. and Jacobs, M. (2003) *Conscious and Unconscious*. Maidenhead: Open University Press.

Erikson, E. (1950) *Childhood and Society*. New York: Norton.

Fairbairn, W.R.D. (1952) *Psychoanalytic Studies of the Personality*. London: Routledge.

Field, N. (1996) *Breakdown and Breakthrough*. London: Routledge.

Franz von, M.-L. (2000) *The Problem of the Puer Aeternus*, 3rd edn. Toronto: Inner City Books.

Freud, S. (1894a) 'The Anxiety Neurosis'. *Collected Papers 1*. London: Hogarth Press (1953).

Freud, S. (1899) *The Interpretation of Dreams*. New York: Avon Books.

Freud, S. (1923b) 'A neurosis of demonic possession in the 17th century', *SE* 4. London: Hogarth Press.

Gabarino, J. and Gilliam, G. (1980) *Understanding Abusive Families*. Toronto: Lexington Books.

Hackmann, A. (1997) *The Transformation of Meaning in Psychological Therapies: Integrating Theory and Practice*. Chichester: Wiley.

Hagelin, J. (2006) *The Secret* (DVD). Luxembourg: TS Production LLC.

Hall, J. A. (1986) *The Jungian Experience*. Toronto: Inner City Books.

Hillman, J. (1996) *The Soul's Code*. London: Bantam Books.

Hycner, R. (1993) *Between Person and Person: Toward a Dialogical Psychotherapy*. New York: Gestalt Journal Press.

Jung, C.G. (1995) *Memories, Dreams, Reflections*. London: Fontana Press.

Krishnamurti, J. (1987) *The Awakening of Intelligence*. London: HarperCollins.

Lowen, A. (1958) *The Language of the Body*. New York: Collier.

Lowen, A. (1975) *Bioenergetics*. Harmondsworth: Penguin.

Madeley, R. (2009) *Fathers & Sons*. London: Simon & Schuster.

March-Smith, R. (2005) *Counselling Skills for Complementary Therapists*. Maidenhead: Open University Press.

Millenson, J.R. (1982) *Mind Matters: Psychological Medicine in Holistic Practice*. Seattle: Eastland Press.

Nupen, C. (2009) *Pyotr Ilyich Tchaikovsky* (DVD). Guildford: Allegro Films.

Perera, S.B. (1981) *Descent to the Goddess: A Way of Initiation for Women*. Toronto: Inner City Books.

Phillips, A. (1988) *Winnicott*. London: Fontana Press.

Pietroni, P. (1986) *Holistic Living*. London: Dent.

Pirani, A. (1988) *The Absent Father: Crisis and Creativity*. London: Arkana.

Pribram, K. (1982) What the fuss is all about, in K. Wilber (ed.) *The Holographic Paradigm*. New York: Shambhala.

Reber, A.S. (1995). *The Dictionary of Psychology*. London: Penguin/Viking.

Ricard, M. (2010) *The Art of Meditation*. New York: Atlantic Books.

Rogers, C. (1961) *On Becoming a Person*. London: Constable.

Rowan, J. (1983) *The Reality Game: A Guide to Humanistic Councelling and Therapy*. London: Routledge and Kegan Paul.

Schutz, W. (1967) *Joy. Expanding Human Awareness*. New York: Grove Press.

Slater-Walker, G. and C. (2002) *An Asperger Marriage*. London: Jessica Kingsley Publishers.

Stein, R. (1973) *Incest and Human Love*. Dallas: Spring Publications.

Stolorow, R.D. (2007) *Trauma and Human Existence*. New York: Analytic Press.

Tantam, D. (1988) Lifelong eccentricity and social isolation: Asperger's syndrome or schizoid personality disorder?, *British Journal of Psychiatry* 153: 783–91.

Temoshok, L. and Dreher, H. (1992) *The Type C Connection: The Behavioral Links to Cancer and Your Health*. New York: Random House.

Walker, M. (1992) *Surviving Secrets*. Buckingham: Open University Press.

Winnicott, D.W. (1974) Fear of breakdown, *Internal Review of Psycho-Analysis*, 1: 103–7.

Winnicott, D.W. (1986) *Home Is Where We Start From*. New York: Norton.

Woodman, M. (1990) *The Ravaged Bridegroom*. Toronto: Inner City Books.

Index

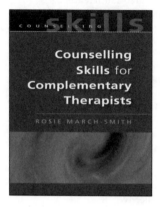

**COUNSELLING SKILLS FOR
COMPLEMENTARY THERAPISTS**

Rosie March-Smith

ISBN (Paperback) 9780335211227
2005

eBook also available

As the demand for tighter professionalism grows in the complementary
healing world, and government regulation increases, a more skilled
approach to counselling patients has become priority.

Key features:

- Covers topics such as transference and counter-transference
- Provides case studies, practical tips, personal anecdotes and
  observations
- Identifies the key skills that a complementary therapist should
  develop and how they might be used more effectively

www.openup.co.uk

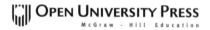

OPEN UNIVERSITY PRESS
McGraw - Hill Education

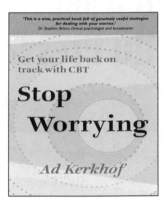

STOP WORRYING
Get Your Life Back on
Track with CBT

Ad Kerkhof

ISBN (Paperback) 9780335242528
2010

eBook also available

This practical book will give you insight into the content, nature and seriousness of your worrying.

Key features:

- Supports and offers advice to worriers
- Contains Cognitive Behavioural Therapy exercises
- Provides guidance for professionals

www.openup.co.uk

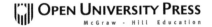

OPEN UNIVERSITY PRESS
McGraw - Hill Education

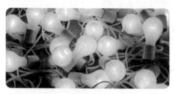 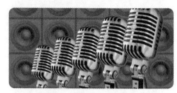
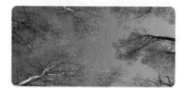 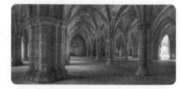
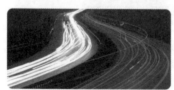 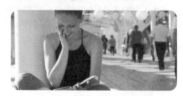
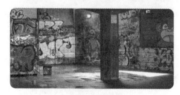
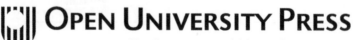